BRAIN REWARD SYSTEMS AND ABUSE

RM
315
.I5375
1985

Brain Reward Systems and Abuse

*Seventh International Berzelius Symposium
Sponsored by the Swedish Society of Medicine*

Editors

Jörgen Engel, M.D., Ph.D.
Professor
Department of Pharmacology
University of Göteborg
Göteborg, Sweden

Lars Oreland, M.D., Ph.D.
Professor
Department of Pharmacology
University of Uppsala
Uppsala, Sweden

David H. Ingvar, M.D., Ph.D.
Professor
President of The Swedish Society of Medicine
1984–1985
Department of Clinical Neurophysiology
University of Lund
Lund, Sweden

Bengt Pernow, M.D., Ph.D.
Professor
Chairman of Berzelius Symposia Committee
President of the Swedish Society of Medicine
1985–1986
Department of Clinical Physiology
Karolinska Hospital
Stockholm, Sweden

Stephan Rössner, M.D., Ph.D.
Associate Professor
King Gustav V Research Institute
Stockholm, Sweden

Lars Åke Pellborn, B.A.
Executive Director
The Swedish Society of Medicine
Stockholm, Sweden

Raven Press New York

Tennessee Tech. Library
Cookeville, Tenn.

368431

Raven Press, 1185 Avenue of the Americas, New York, New York 10036

© 1987 by Raven Press Books, Ltd. All rights reserved. This book is protected by copyright. No part of it may be reproduced, stored in a retrieval system, or transmitted, in any form or by any means, electronic, mechanical, photocopying, recording, or otherwise, without the prior written permission of the publisher.

Made in the United States of America

9 8 7 6 5 4 3 2 1

Library of Congress Cataloging-in-Publication Data

International Berzelius Symposium (7th : 1985 :
    Göteborg, Sweden)
    Brain reward systems and abuse.

    Held at Göteborg, Sweden, Oct. 1985.
    Includes bibliographies and index.
    1. Neuropsychopharmacology—Congresses.
    2. Brain, Effect of drugs on—Congresses.
    3. Reward (Psychology)—Congresses. 4. Drug
    abuse—Physiological aspects. Congresses.
    I. Engel, Jörgen. II. Svenska läkaresäallskapet.
    III. Title. [DNLM: 1. Brain—drug effects—
    congresses. 2. Reward—congresses. 3. Substance
    Abuse—congresses. W3 IN123N 7th 1985b /
    WL 300 I592 1985b]

RM315.I5375   1985   615'.78   85-43233
ISBN 0-88167-263-7

Preface

Since 1984, the Swedish Society of Medicine has organized a series of symposia in honor of the famous Swedish biochemist and physician Jöns Jakob Berzelius (1779–1848), who was one of the founders of our society. These symposia attempt to cover important medical topics with wide social implications. They have been made possible by generous donations from Swedish corporations and organizations who in this way support Swedish medical research and an international exchange of medical scientific information.

Abuse of drugs and alcohol is an enormous problem in most countries. The cerebral mechanisms behind dependence and abuse have previously been and still are poorly understood. The highly important psychological factors have often been in the foreground. Since the last decades, however, animal models and clinical findings have shown that the brain contains "reward systems" (previously termed "pleasure centers") through which the psychological factors operate. It is the morphology and physiology, and indeed pharmacology, of these systems that is the focus of this volume. As the reader will note, current research on the reward systems has opened up several new roads to a deeper understanding of the neuronal machineries that are of especial importance for the experience of pleasure and reward, be it of the "physiological" type caused by food, love, appreciation, achievements etc., or the intense abnormal type elicited by drugs of abuse, including alcohol.

This volume brings together both experimental and clinical workers interested in abuse research.

David H. Ingvar President (1984–85)
of the Swedish Society of Medicine

v

Acknowledgments

In 1983, the Swedish Society of Medicine celebrated its 175th anniversary. This event inspired a fund drive to enable the Society to hold international scientific symposia on important sociomedical problems. The society received many generous and substantial contributions to its 175th anniversary fund. The symposia were named after the famous Swedish biochemist Jöns Jakob Berzelius (1779–1848), who was one of the founders of our society. This symposium on brain reward systems is the seventh Berzelius Symposium. Other symposia have dealt with, e.g., drug effects on the brain, brain injuries due to boxing, and alcohol and the developing brain.

The symposium on which this volume is based was made possible by a special and very generous grant from Sven and Dagmar Sahlén Foundation. On behalf of the Swedish Society of Medicine, sincere thanks are expressed to the Foundation for this aid.

The Society would also like to thank Drs. Jörgen Engel and Lars Oreland, who carried the great burden of organizing the meeting. The chancellary and technical staff, especially Ms. May Hedqvist of the Society, are thanked for their help with the arrangements.

The Swedish Society of Medicine expresses its sincere thanks to all the prominent researchers from the international and national scenes who participated and who enabled the ensuing overview of one of the most important sociomedical field today.

Contents

Contributors

Marianne Amalric
*Division of Preclinical Neuroscience and
    Endocrinology
Scripps Clinic and Research Foundation
10666 North Torrey Pines Road
La Jolla, California 92037*

Burton Angrist
*Department of Psychiatry
New York University Medical Center and
Veterans Administration Medical Center
First Avenue at East 24th Street
New York, New York 10010*

Nils Bejerot
*Department of Social Medicine
Karolinska Institute
S-172 83 Sundbyberg, Sweden*

James D. Belluzzi
*Department of Pharmacology
College of Medicine
University of California at Irvine
Irvine, California 92717*

Floyd E. Bloom
*Division of Preclinical Neuroscience and
    Endocrinology
Scripps Clinic and Research Foundation
10666 North Torrey Pines Road
La Jolla, California 92037*

Stefan Borg
*Department of Psychiatry
Karolinska Institute
St. Göran's Hospital
S-112 81 Stockholm, Sweden*

Michael A. Bozarth
*Department of Psychology
Center for Studies in Behavioral
    Neurobiology
Concordia University
Montreal, Quebec H3G 1M8, Canada*

Hans Christian Fibiger
*Division of Neurological Sciences
Department of Psychiatry
University of British Columbia
Vancouver, B.C., V6T 1W5, Canada*

Robert Freedman
*Department of Psychiatry
University of Colorado Health Sciences
    Center
4200 East 9th Avenue
Denver, Colorado 80262*

Jack E. Henningfield
*National Institute on Drug Abuse
P.O. Box 5180
Baltimore, Maryland 21224*

Barry J. Hoffer
*Department of Pharmacology, C-236
University of Colorado Health Sciences
    Center
4200 East 9th Avenue
Denver, Colorado 80262*

Paula L. Hoffman
*National Institute on Alcohol Abuse and
    Alcoholism
Laboratory for Studies of Neuroadaptive
    Processes
National Institutes of Health
12501 Washington Avenue
Rockville, Maryland 20852*

Jerome H. Jaffe
*National Institute on Drug Abuse
Addiction Research Center
P.O. Box 5180
Baltimore, Maryland 21224*

George F. Koob
*Division of Preclinical Neuroscience and
    Endocrinology
Scripps Clinic and Research Foundation
10666 North Torrey Pines Road
La Jolla, California 92037*

Mary O. Lawrin
Clinical Pharmacology Program
Addiction Research Foundation
33 Russell Street
Toronto, Ontario M5S 2S1, Canada

Paula Liljeberg
Department of Psychiatry
Karolinksa Institute
St. Göran's Hospital
S-112 81 Stockholm, Sweden

Edythe D. London
National Institute on Drug Abuse
Addiction Research Center
P.O. Box 5180
Baltimore, Maryland 21224

Dick Mossberg
Department of Psychiatry
Karolinska Institute
St. Göran's Hospital
S-112 81 Stockholm, Sweden

Claudio A. Naranjo
Clinical Pharmacology Program
Addiction Research Foundation
33 Russell Street
Toronto, Ontario M5S 2S1, Canada

Michael R. Palmer
Department of Pharmacology, C-236
University of Colorado Health Sciences
Center
4200 East 9th Avenue
Denver, Colorado 80262

A. G. Phillips
Division of Neurological Sciences
Department of Psychology
University of British Columbia
Vancouver, B.C., V6T 1W5, Canada

Linda J. Porrino
Laboratory of Cerebral Metabolism
National Institute of Mental Health
36/1A-05, 9000 Rockville Pike
Bethesda, Maryland 20892

Edward M. Sellers
Clinical Pharmacology Program
Addiction Research Foundation
33 Russell Street
Toronto, Ontario M5S 2S1, Canada

Larry Stein
Department of Pharmacology
College of Medicine
University of California at Irvine
Irvine, California 92717

John T. Sullivan
Clinical Pharmacology Program
Addiction Research Foundation
33 Russell Street
Toronto, Ontario M5S 2S1, Canada

Boris Tabakoff
National Institute on Alcohol Abuse and
Alcoholism
National Institutes of Health Clinical
Center
Bldg. 10, Room 3C103
Bethesda, Maryland 20205

Jan M. Van Ree
Rudolf Magnus Institute for
Pharmacology
Medical Faculty
University of Utrecht
Vondellaan 6
3521 GD Utrecht, The Netherlands

Franco Vaccarino
Division of Preclinical Neuroscience and
Endocrinology
Scripps Clinic and Research Foundation
10666 North Torrey Pines Road
La Jolla, California 92037

Yun Wang
Department of Pharmacology
University of Colorado Health Sciences
Center
4200 East 9th Avenue
Denver, Colorado 80262

Marvin Zuckerman
Department of Psychology
University of Delaware
Newark, Delaware 19716

Brain Reward Systems and Abuse, edited by
J. Engel and L. Oreland.
Raven Press, New York © 1987.

Ventral Tegmental Reward System

Michael A. Bozarth

*Department of Psychology, Center for Studies in Behavioral Neurobiology, Concordia
University, Montreal, Quebec H3G 1M8, Canada*

Several brain functions appear to have specialized systems that mediate their actions. The visual and auditory systems are two systems that have distinct neural pathways involved in the processing of their information. Some other brain functions seem to involve more diffuse systems, such as those involved in learning and memory. The notion that motivational processes may involve specialized brain circuitry received its first empirical support from the pioneering work of Hess (33), who showed that electrical stimulation of certain brain regions elicited behaviors that were highly organized and complex. The demonstration that specialized brain circuitry can control large segments of complex behaviors opened the possibility that similar systems might be identified for other motivated behaviors, such as feeding and drinking.

There are several approaches to the study of brain mechanisms involved in motivation and reward. One approach is to observe behavior and measure changes in CNS activity that accompany specific behaviors. This correlational approach has been used to study the neural basis of a number of behaviors. One can attempt to identify neurochemical changes that are associated with a certain behavior; alternatively, anatomical relationships can be inferred through the use of electrophysiological recordings that determine which pathways are active during specific behaviors.

Another approach that has been used to study brain systems mediating behavior is a functional approach. Here, the activity of specific brain systems can be manipulated to determine their influence on behavior. The activity of these pathways can be stimulated either electrically or chemically, or the function of these systems can be disrupted through the use of selective lesioning procedures. Essentially, the functional role of these brain systems is explored (a) by causing the appearance of the behavior through stimulation and (b) by blocking the behavior by selectively eliminating the activity of a specific brain region.

The functional approach asks two related but nonetheless different questions: Is the activity of a given brain region sufficient to produce the behavior in question? Is the activity of a given brain region necessary to produce the behavior in question? Frequently, the activity of a brain system may be both a sufficient and a necessary condition for a given behavior to occur. There is, however, no reason

1

to suspect that these two conditions should always be satisfied by the same brain systems.

BRAIN STIMULATION REWARD

The early reports that rats would work to electrically stimulate certain parts of their brains (40,42) were very exciting and seemed to suggest that a specialized brain system may mediate reward function. Subsequent studies, however, soon showed that many different electrode placements supported brain stimulation reward and that this phenomenon was not restricted to a single focus. Nonetheless, electrode placements in the lateral hypothalamic level of the medial forebrain bundle and in the ventral tegmental area seemed to produce the strongest indication of reward, and attempts were made to functionally link these areas with the various brain sites supporting brain stimulation reward (e.g., ref. 41).

Dopamine Link

The common denominator that appeared to link the various electrode placements was the catecholamine systems in the brain (27). With the finding that disruption of catecholamine synthesis blocked the rewarding effect of electrical stimulation, the catecholamine hypothesis was thrust to the forefront (17,57). Further studies examined the relative importance of norepinephrine and dopamine in brain stimulation reward and revealed that dopaminergic mechanisms were primarily responsible for the rewarding action of electrical stimulation. In addition, a number of tests have been developed to distinguish reward from motoric deficits following dopamine-receptor blockade (23,24).

The rewarding impact of electrical stimulation, at least from some electrode placements such as those in the lateral hypothalamic area, depends on the integrity of brain dopamine systems (21,22,66,67). The blockade of dopamine receptors disrupts the rewarding effects of this electrical stimulation, whereas drugs that augment dopaminergic neurotransmission appear to enhance brain stimulation reward. The effects of dopamine-depleting lesions are less clear, with some investigators reporting a disruption of self-stimulation (14,22,36), whereas others find little enduring effect (14,31). The reported failures to disrupt brain stimulation reward with dopamine-depleting lesions are probably related to inadequate dopamine depletions. Much of the research has focused on the ventral tegmental dopamine system with its cell bodies in the ventral tegmental area and with ascending projections terminating in several brain regions, including the nucleus accumbens and the frontal cortex, although some evidence suggests that the nigrostriatal dopamine system may also be involved in rewarding brain stimulation.

First-Stage Neurons

Although the evidence seems compelling that dopamine plays a critical role in brain stimulation, recent data suggest that the neurons directly activated by the electrical stimulation are not, in fact, dopamine neurons. Through an elegant series of experiments, Shizgal and colleagues have shown that the electrophysiological properties of the neurons directly driven by rewarding brain stimulation (i.e., the first-stage neurons) have characteristics not found in dopaminergic neurons. The actual procedure used to study the electrophysiological properties of the neurons directly activated by brain stimulation reward is complex (26,54), but the conceptual basis of this approach is relatively simple.

If a neuron is stimulated by a suprathreshold stimulus, an action potential is generated as in Fig. 1A. If a second stimulation pulse is delivered during the

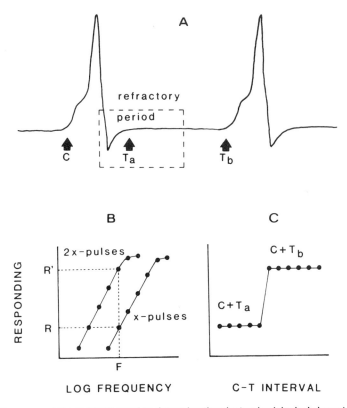

FIG. 1. Summary of the methods used to determine the electrophysiological characteristics of neurons involved in brain stimulation reward. Although the illustration represents an oversimplification of the actual procedures used, the conceptual basis of this work is relatively simple. See text for a description. This figure is developed from the work of Gallistel et al. (26), Shizgal and colleagues (2,52,54), and Yeomans (72).

refractory period (T_a), then the second stimulation pulse will be ineffective, and only one action potential is produced. If, however, the second pulse (T_b) is delivered after the refractory period, then two action potentials will be generated by the pair of stimulation pulses. The minimum interval between the conditioning pulse (C) and the test pulse (T) that produces two action potentials is dependent on the refractory period of the neuron. Behaviorally, the performance of an animal receiving rewarding brain stimulation is related to the frequency of that stimulation. Within a certain range of values, performance will increase as a function of stimulation frequency or the number of pulses delivered during each train of stimulation. Figure 1B shows the effect of doubling the number of pulses in each stimulation train that an animal receives. Note that doubling the number of pulses shifts the frequency response curve to the left, indicating that the effectiveness of the stimulation has increased. For example, an animal stimulated at frequency F with x pulses will respond at level R in Fig. 1B. If the animal receives $2x$ pulses, then stimulation frequency F would be associated with performance level R'. If a series of pulse pairs is delivered with various intervals between the conditioning pulse and the test pulse ($C-T$ interval), the test pulse in some $C-T$ intervals will fall within the neuron's refractory period ($C + T_a$), whereas other test pulses will occur after the refractory period ($C + T_b$). $C-T$ intervals that are longer than the refractory period of the stimulated neuron will produce an abrupt shift in responding, as shown in Figure 1C, indicating that the animal is responding to $2x$ rather than x pulses of rewarding stimulation. This procedure can be used to estimate the refractory period of neurons directly activated by rewarding brain stimulation.

A direct adaptation of this method can be used to determine anatomical connections and conduction velocities of the first-stage neurons. This procedure delivers the conditioning pulse and the test pulse through two different electrodes. If the electrodes are stimulating the same set of neurons, then stimulation with $C-T$ intervals that are within the refractory period result in only the conditioning pulse of the stimulation pulse pairs being effective in triggering action potentials. When the test pulses are ineffective in producing action potentials, a collision has occured (see refs. 26 and 54), and the animal's performance is based on the rewarding effect of only the conditioning pulses. If the $C-T$ interval is longer than the refractory period and the time necessary for the action potential to travel between the two electrodes, then the pulse pairs will produce an abrupt change in performance, indicating that both the conditioning and test pulses are effective in initiating action potentials. This procedure tests for collision between the two pulses delivered through different electrodes and can thus determine if the two electrodes are stimulating the same fiber system. Furthermore, conduction velocity estimates can be derived by subtracting the refractory period from the minimum $C-T$ interval required to produce the higher level of performance and then dividing this time by the distance between the two electrodes.

These studies have clearly shown that the conduction velocities of neurons directly activated by rewarding brain stimulation are much faster than those of catecholamine neurons (2,54). In fact, the conduction velocity estimates (1 to 8 meters/sec) suggest that the first-stage neurons are fast-conducting, myelinated fibers. Furthermore, because a collision effect can be shown between lateral hypothalamic and ventral tegmental electrode placements, this research suggests that the rewarding signal travels without synaptic interruption between these two brain regions (52,54). Finally, work using an anodal block technique, adapted from classic electrophysiological studies, suggests that the direction of conduction is from lateral hypothalamus to ventral tegmentum (53).

The work of Shizgal and co-workers has ruled out dopamine neurons as the fibers directly activated by rewarding brain stimulation. Nonetheless, brain dopamine systems do seem to play a critical role in brain stimulation reward, and the possibility remains that the first-stage neurons make synaptic contact with the ventral tegmental dopamine system. Thus, electrical stimulation could trans-synaptically activate an ascending dopamine system. This would appear to be among the simplest hypotheses integrating the pharmacological and anatomical data with the electrophysiological data. Other possibilities, however, are equally viable.

Dopamine Hypothesis Revisited

If dopamine systems are activated by rewarding stimulation of the lateral hypothalamus, then the activity of the ascending dopamine systems should be increased by rewarding stimulation. There are several methods that could be used to determine the effect of brain stimulation reward on various neural systems. One method uses the uptake of radiolabeled glucose as an index of general cell activity (55). Neurons that are activated by rewarding brain stimulation should show an increased uptake of glucose that can be detected with autoradiography.

Esposito et al. (20) have shown that ventral tegmental stimulation produces an increase in glucose uptake (and presumably in cell activity) in a number of brain systems including elements that correspond to the trajectory of the ventral tegmental dopamine system. This study supports the notion that electrical stimulation in the region of the ventral tegmentum can activate brain dopamine systems. Other studies using dopamine metabolite formation as an index of dopamine activity have shown a similar increase in activity of the nigrostriatal dopamine system following electrical stimulation of the substantia nigra (39,70).

Although these lines of evidence are very encouraging, they really have little significance to the question of whether lateral hypothalamic stimulation activates dopaminergic neurons. Electrodes placed directly in the dopamine cell body regions may be capable of activating these dopamine systems, but this does not determine if rewarding stimulation of the first-stage neurons (known not to be dopaminergic) similarly activates ascending dopamine neurons.

Gallistel and co-workers (25,71) have assessed changes in brain metabolic activity following rewarding lateral hypothalamic stimulation. Their studies have failed to reveal an activation of brain dopamine systems, although there is a clear activation of some neural system that appears to connect with the ventral tegmentum (possibly the first-stage neurons). A number of factors could account for a failure to demonstrate the activation of dopamine systems. One obvious possibility is that this method is not sensitive to the activation of relatively small-fiber-diameter neurons such as those in the dopamine systems. However, subsequent work has shown that direct electrical stimulation of the substantia nigra, which is known to activate brain dopamine systems (39,70), produces a marked increase in glucose uptake in neurons that topographically correspond to the nigrostriatal dopamine system (25). Similarly, neuroleptic treatment, which also increases dopaminergic activity, produces an increase in glucose uptake in brain regions corresponding to the nigrostriatal and ventral tegmental dopamine systems (25), although the increase is less than might be predicted on the basis of neurochemical evidence. Thus, this method would appear to be sensitive to changes in the activity of these dopaminergic systems. Even so, the large number of cells activated by electrical stimulation might mask the enhanced activity of a relatively small dopaminergic system. Electrical stimulation is nonspecific in activating most neurons proximal to the electrode tip; in addition, motor pathways involved in lever-pressing should also show an increase in metabolic activity. These effects could easily obscure an increase in the metabolic activity of the relatively small dopamine systems.

Another approach to determining the effects of rewarding stimulation on brain dopamine systems is to directly measure the effects of this stimulation on dopamine systems. Preliminary data suggest that lateral hypothalamic stimulation produces a net reduction in brain dopamine levels in both the ventral tegmentum and the nucleus accumbens (M. Bozarth, *unpublished observations*, 1985). In this study, several groups of rats were allowed to lever-press for brain stimulation reward for 1 hr at one of three stimulation intensities. At the end of this period, animals were immediately sacrificed by decapitation and the brains rapidly removed. High-performance liquid chromatography revealed a depletion of dopamine in the ventral tegmental area and in the nucleus accumbens. Figure 2 shows the extent of nucleus accumbens dopamine depletions as a function of stimulation intensity. Similar effects were seen on the contralateral side, except that the lowest stimulation intensity did not produce any significant reductions. Although the exact cause of this reduction in dopamine is not known, it seems likely that activation of the ventral tegmental dopamine system by rewarding lateral hypothalamic stimulation produced this depletion. The magnitude of dopamine release probably exceeded the synthesis rate of these neurons. In partial support of this explanation, a reliable increase in homovanillic acid/dopamine ratios was observed. These data suggest that the ventral tegmental dopamine system is, in fact, activated by rewarding stimulation of the lateral hypothalamus. It is interesting to note that the stimulation parameters used in this study were very similar to those that Gallistel and colleagues (25,71) found ineffective in producing increased glucose uptake in neurons anatomically corresponding to

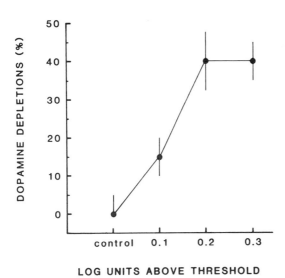

FIG. 2. Decreases in dopamine levels following rewarding stimulation of the lateral hypothalamic area. Current intensity thresholds were determined using a two-lever autotitration method (4). Animals self-stimulated for 1 hr at a fixed current intensity ranging from 0.1 to 0.3 log units above their thresholds. Decreases in dopamine levels as a function of stimulation intensity are illustrated for the nucleus accumbens ipsilateral to the stimulating electrode. Similar effects were seen on the contralateral side, except the lowest stimulation intensity produced no change in dopamine levels. Note that the bilateral activation seen in the present study with lateral hypothalamic stimulation parallels the bilateral activation reported by Esposito et al. (20) following ventral tegmental stimulation.

the ventral tegmental dopamine system. Considerably more work needs to be done to fully understand this effect.

DRUG REINFORCEMENT

Traditionally, theories of drug addiction have stressed the role of preexisting factors in the acquisition of an addiction. These factors included such things as addictive personalities, psychological stress, or even genetic theories based in part on biological explanations. Some drugs, such as the opiates, were presumed to be addictive because of their ability to relieve the aversive consequences of withdrawal. Although these theories still enjoy some popularity, many investigators have shifted their attention to a different dimension of the actions of these addictive drugs—their ability to directly reinforce behavior. A consensus is developing among many workers in the field of drug addiction suggesting that addictive drugs are taken because of their ability to pharmacologically activate brain systems involved in reinforcement.

Interactions with Brain Stimulation Reward

Addictive drugs have pronounced effects on brain stimulation reward. Drugs such as the psychomotor stimulants (e.g., amphetamine, cocaine) and opiates (e.g., morphine, heroin, methadone) appear to enhance the rewarding effects of electrical brain stimulation. This facilitation effect is demonstrable as an increase in pressing rates for fixed intensity stimulation (45) or as a lowering of current intensity (19) and frequency (50) thresholds for brain stimulation reward. Similar effects have been reported for both measures of performance for rewarding electrical stimulation. In addition to the opiates and psychomotor stimulants, barbiturates and ethanol can facilitate brain stimulation reward (67). On the other hand, drugs with a low addiction potential generally fail to facilitate brain stimulation reward. This relationship suggests that facilitation of brain stimulation reward may reflect a drug's intrinsic rewarding action. Furthermore, these data provided the first evidence for an important interaction between addictive drugs and brain reward systems.

Study of Drugs as Reinforcers

Another approach to studying the rewarding properties of drugs involves directly studying their ability to reinforce behavior. Animals can be trained to lever-press in order to receive intravenous injections of most drugs that are addictive in humans (29,63,73). Furthermore, laboratory animals generally do not self-administer drugs that are not addictive in humans. The study of drugs as reinforcers provides a direct method of assessing drug reinforcement and a method to study the interaction of addictive drugs with brain reward systems. Furthermore, addictive drugs generally control behavior in much the same manner as conventional reinforcers such as food and water (56). With this perspective, the study of drug addiction focuses on the study of drugs as reinforcers and becomes a simple extension of basic operant psychology.

The study of the neural substrates involved in drug reinforcement has frequently used intravenous self-administration techniques. Animals can be trained to self-administer a drug, and the effects of lesions of various brain regions on drug-taking can be examined (49). Similarly, brain lesions can be made, and the effects on the acquisition of drug-taking can be evaluated. Both of these approaches attempt to identify brain regions that are necessary for drug reward. Another method that has recently been used to identify brain areas involved in drug reward uses a modification of intravenous self-administration methods: cannulae can be implanted into brain tissue and animals trained to self-administer drug directly into discrete brain regions (3). This method attempts to identify brain areas where drug application is sufficient to reinforce behavior. The neural elements responsible for the initiation of the rewarding action of a drug can thus be localized.

Psychomotor Stimulant Reward

Psychomotor stimulant drugs have strong actions on catecholamine systems. Cocaine blocks the reuptake of catecholamines (32), and amphetamine releases stored catecholamines and blocks their reuptake (1,15); these actions significantly enhance the activity of both dopamine and norepinephrine. Early work using pharmacological challenges of intravenous stimulant self-administration revealed the importance of dopaminergic neurotransmission in the rewarding action of these drugs (74,75). Drugs that selectively block dopamine receptors caused a change in the pattern of drug intake that resembled the effect of decreasing the amount of drug given per injection. Low to moderate doses of a dopamine-receptor blocking drug increased stimulant self-administration, whereas higher doses caused an extinction pattern of responding similar to that seen when drug vehicle is substituted for the reinforcing drug injections. Drugs that blocked norepinephrine receptors failed to produce these characteristic changes in responding for drug. Thus, whereas stimulants activate both dopaminergic and noradrenergic systems, only the dopaminergic action is critical to the rewarding impact of these drugs. This has led to the notion that enhanced dopaminergic activity produces reward (67). Furthermore, this work illustrates the importance of functional studies of brain reward systems. Because psychomotor stimulants increase both noradrenergic and dopaminergic activity, correlative neurochemistry might have suggested that both catecholamines were involved in stimulant reward. However, the effect of selective norepinephrine- and dopamine-receptor blockers clearly shows that only dopaminergic activity is essential for psychomotor stimulant reward.

The brain region critically involved in psychomotor stimulant reward has also been identified. Dopamine-depleting lesions in the nucleus accumbens disrupt intravenous amphetamine and cocaine self-administration (37,46,48). Lesions of other dopamine terminal fields (e.g., caudate nucleus) or of noradrenergic systems do not affect stimulant self-administration (49). On the other hand, lesions of the cell body region of the ventral tegmental dopamine system effectively disrupt intravenous stimulant self-administration (47). Further corroboration of the rewarding action of stimulants in this dopamine system comes from a study showing the direct intracranial self-administration of amphetamine into the nucleus accumbens (34; but see ref. 43). Taken together, these data suggest that the rewarding impact of stimulant drugs is mediated by the ventral tegmental dopamine system.

Opiate Reward

Because of the importance of the ventral tegmental dopamine system in psychomotor stimulant reward, this system is an obvious candidate for the neural substrate mediating opiate reward. The data suggest that activation of the ventral tegmental dopamine system is rewarding, and if opiates could activate this system, this activation should also be rewarding. Furthermore, the facilitatory action of morphine on brain stimulation reward has been localized to cells in the ventral tegmental area (12,13), and this suggests that opiates may, in fact, activate this important system involved in motivation and reward.

The effects of opiates on dopamine systems are not as clear as those of psychomotor stimulants on these systems. Some investigators have suggested that opiates actually inhibit dopaminergic neurotransmission (18,51) and even that opiate reward involves an attenuation of brain dopamine function (28). It seems surprising, however, that a class of drugs with such potent reinforcing effects would inhibit a brain system that is involved in brain stimulation reward and in the rewarding effects of psychomotor stimulants.

The microinjection of morphine into the ventral tegmental area produces contralateral rotation (3,7,35), indicative of enhanced dopaminergic neurotransmission (59). Furthermore, the cell firing rates of dopamine-containing cells in the ventral tegmentum are increased by both the systemic and microiontophoretic application of morphine (30,38). Direct evidence for the ability of morphine to enhance dopaminergic neurotransmission comes from neurochemical studies showing that accumbens 3-methoxytyramine levels are increased following morphine injections (64,69). Because this dopamine metabolite appears to index the activity of released dopamine (16,65,69), this line of evidence is particularly compelling.

Animals will readily learn a lever-pressing response to self-administer opiates directly into the ventral tegmental area (6,62). As shown in Fig. 3, other brain areas do not appear to support the rapid acquisition seen with ventral tegmental morphine injections (3,7). Dopamine-depleting lesions of the ventral tegmental dopamine system disrupt the acquisition of intravenous heroin self-administration (10); the same lesions do not affect responding for food reinforcement,

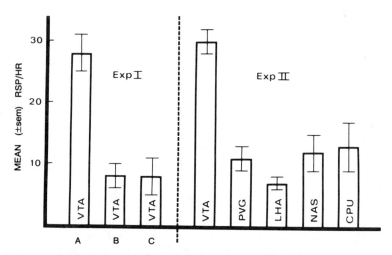

FIG. 3. Intracranial self-administration of morphine. The *first panel* shows intracranial morphine (100 ng/infusion) self-administration into the ventral tegmental area (Group A), a yoked control (Group B) where animals passively received intracranial morphine injections but were not allowed to self-administer the drug, and a vehicle control (Group C). The *second panel* shows the results of an anatomical mapping study. Intracranial morphine self-administration was seen in the ventral tegmental area (VTA) but not in the periventricular gray area (PVG), the lateral hypothalamic area (LHA), the nucleus accumbens (NAS), or the caudate nucleus (CPU). (From Bozarth and Wise, ref. 7, with permission.)

indicating that this effect is not the result of an impairment in performance or learning (10). Furthermore, drugs that block dopamine receptors attenuate the rewarding effects of opiates (5,44). In addition, there is some evidence that an opiate action in the nucleus accumbens may also be rewarding (61), although controversy exists regarding the relative importance of this action in comparison with the opiate action in the ventral tegmentum area (cf. refs. 11 and 60).

It is particularly interesting to note that the rewarding action of morphine applied in the ventral tegmental area does not involve physiological dependence (9). A popular explanation of opiate addiction focuses on the motivational properties of withdrawal discomfort and the ability of opiates to relieve this distress. Drug taking is seen as being under the control of a negative reinforcement process, whereby the primary motivation to take the drug is governed by its ability to relieve withdrawal discomfort. The intracranial self-administration of morphine is not accompanied by any signs of physical dependence (9). Furthermore, continuous infusions of morphine into the ventral tegmentum fail to produce physical dependence, whereas similar infusions into the periventricular gray area produce strong physical dependence (9). Thus, the rewarding action of ventral tegmental morphine is independent of physical dependence mechanisms.

Another technique has provided direct evidence for the partial cross-substitution of psychomotor stimulant and opiate rewards. Animals lever-pressing for intravenous drug will show a pause in their drug intake if a noncontingent injection of that drug is given (73). That is, if an animal is intravenously self-administering cocaine, a noncontingent, experimenter-delivered injection of cocaine will produce a pause in the subject's self-administered drug intake. This is probably related to the regulation of drug intake that is well established for psychomotor stimulants (73). The fact that noncontingent drug reward can cause

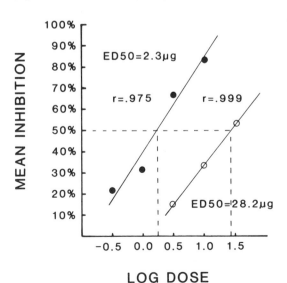

FIG. 4. The effect of ventral tegmental morphine injections on intravenous cocaine self-administration (1 mg/kg/infusion). Morphine microinjections were unilateral, and the doses are indicated on the abscissa. The figure shows the inhibition of cocaine intake 1 to 2 hr after central morphine injections. Dose–response data were obtained with (*open circles*) and without (*filled circles*) systemic naltrexone pretreatment (3 mg/kg). (From Bozarth and Wise, ref. 10, with permission.)

a change in self-administered drug intake provides a particularly interesting test for the hypothesis that opiates and psychomotor stimulants may activate the same brain reward system. As shown in Fig. 4, ventral tegmental morphine injections cause a dose-dependent decrease in responding for intravenous cocaine injections (10). This change in cocaine intake is predicted from the hypothesis that nucleus accumbens dopamine is released by a morphine action in the ventral tegmental area. Furthermore, the slowing of drug intake is frequently accompanied by increased activity and by responding on an inactive lever, suggesting that a sedative influence of morphine cannot explain this effect. Finally, the fact that systemic narcotic antagonist (i.e., naltrexone) administration produces a parallel shift in the dose–response curve for morphine's inhibition of cocaine intake indicates that the central morphine effect is dependent on the activation of opiate receptors and not the result of some nonspecific, physicochemical action (3).

OVERVIEW OF BRAIN REWARD SYSTEMS

Of the several approaches to the study of brain reward systems, the functional approach identifying individual units involved in reward processes has perhaps been the most fruitful. Most correlative data have been supportive of the hypotheses generated by the functional analyses, although correlative studies alone fail to rule out the involvement of many more brain systems. The determination of what constitutes a necessary condition for reward has also been very informative. In some cases, the identification of the sufficient condition has corresponded to what constitutes a necessary condition, but there are also cases where this relationship does not exist. Nonetheless, a model reward system has been developed using this functional approach, and several anatomical and neurochemical elements have been identified.

A reward system has been delineated that (a) is capable of reinforcing behavior, (b) is dopamine-dependent, (c) anatomically corresponds to the ventral tegmental dopamine system, (d) involves approach behavior, and (e) is activated by (i) lateral hypothalamic electrical stimulation, (ii) psychomotor stimulant drugs, and (iii) opiate drugs. The data suggest that a dopaminergic action in the nucleus accumbens is critical for reward in this system. The identified links in this system include a descending, fast-conducting fiber system that is activated by electrical stimulation; the nucleus accumbens, which is the target of psychomotor stimulant reward; and the ventral tegmentum, which initiates a rewarding action of opiates (Fig. 5). Although other brain systems may also be involved in reward from these events, activation of the ventral tegmental system appears to be a sufficient and possibly a necessary condition for reward from these stimuli. It is likely that other systems are involved in the long-term reinforcing impact of systemic opiate injections; the periventricular gray system is one possible candidate (8). However, the evidence clearly shows that these three diverse rewarding events can all activate

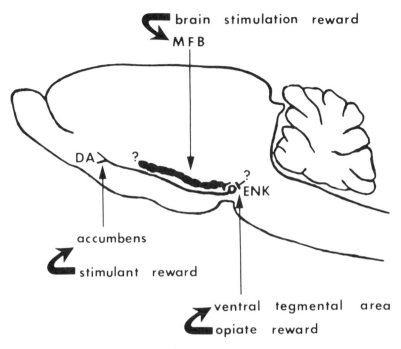

FIG. 5. Proposed brain reward circuitry. Because the thresholds for activation of myelinated fibers are much lower than those for dopaminergic fibers, brain stimulation reward probably does not directly activate the dopamine system with the stimulation parameters normally used. This is consistent with the suggestion that the directly activated neurons are not dopaminergic. However, it is likely that descending, myelinated neurons within the medial forebrain bundle (MFB) trans-synaptically activate the ascending dopamine system. The origin of the descending, myelinated neurons has not been established, but Shizgal et al. (54) suggest several possibilities including the diagonal band of Broca and the bed nucleus of the stria terminalis. The sites where psychomotor stimulants and opiates can activate this reward system are also illustrated. The ventral tegmental action of opiates probably involves an enkephalinergic system (ENK), but the anatomical location of that system has not yet been identified.

the same brain reward system and that such activation is a sufficient condition for the control of behavior (i.e., positive reinforcement).

The question of how many reward systems are involved in the control of behavior remains an open one. Certainly, there are reasons to suspect that multiple brain reward systems exist. Not only are many different behaviors likely to be under the control of different reward systems, but even a single class of behaviors may involve several reward systems. Opiate reward, for example, appears to be mediated primarily by the ventral tegmental dopamine system, but it is likely that physical dependence mechanisms mediated outside of the ventral tegmentum may also be capable of controlling behavior (8) although to a lesser extent than the ventral tegmental system. Once physical dependence has been established by an opiate action in the periventricular gray region, then abstinence from drug will result in withdrawal symptoms, and this aversive condition will be capable of motivating behavior. Because drug intake can relieve the discomfort associated with this withdrawal state, drug-taking behavior would be supported by a negative reinforcement process.

Existing data argue for at least three brain reward systems: a ventral tegmental dopamine system involved in positive reinforcement and approach behavior, a periventricular gray system involved in negative reinforcement and avoidance behavior (8), and a nigrostriatal system involved in the regulation of food and water intake (58). It is interesting to note that even though the functional integrity of the ventral tegmental system is apparently not a necessary condition for the regulation of feeding (i.e., dopamine-depleting lesions of this system fail to disrupt food intake), opiate action in the ventral tegmentum is clearly capable of modulating feeding behavior (68). Thus, feeding is probably under the control of more than one system, and interactions between these systems may exist. There is clearly a difference between neural activation that is sufficient for food reward and neural activation that is necessary for food reward.

The ventral tegmental reward system is probably the best understood of the several proposed brain reward systems. The systematic identification of functional linkages in this reward system has shown that the rewarding impact of several distinct events are, at least in part, mediated by this system. It is particularly tempting to speculate that even more rewarding events may involve the activation of this system. Further studies identifying the neural inputs and outputs of this system and determining the impact of other rewarding stimuli on this system are needed to clearly establish the importance of the ventral tegmental system in the control of other motivated behaviors.

REFERENCES

1. Axelrod, J. (1970): Amphetamine: Metabolism, physiological disposition and its effects on catecholamine storage. In: *Amphetamine and Related Compounds,* edited by E. Costa and S. Garattini, pp. 207–216. Raven Press, New York.
2. Bielajew, C., and Shizgal, P. (1982): Behaviorally derived measures of conduction velocity in the substrate for rewarding medial forebrain bundle stimulation. *Brain Res.,* 237:107–119.
3. Bozarth, M. A. (1983): Opiate reward mechanisms mapped by intracranial self-administration. In: *Neurobiology of Opiate Reward Processes,* edited by J. E. Smith and J. D. Lane, pp. 331–359. Elsevier/North Holland Biomedical Press, Amsterdam.
4. Bozarth, M. A., Gerber, G. J., and Wise, R. A. (1980): Intracranial self-stimulation as a technique to study the rewarding properties of drugs of abuse. *Pharmacol. Biochem. Behav.,* 13(Suppl. 1): 245–247.
5. Bozarth, M. A., and Wise, R. A. (1981): Heroin reward is dependent on a dopaminergic substrate. *Life Sci.,* 29:1881–1886.
6. Bozarth, M. A., and Wise, R. A. (1981): Intracranial self-administration of morphine into the ventral tegmental area. *Life Sci.,* 28:551–555.
7. Bozarth, M. A., and Wise, R. A. (1982): Localization of the reward-relevant opiate receptors. In: *Problems of Drug Dependence, 1981,* edited by L. S. Harris, pp. 158–164. U.S. Government Printing Office, Washington, D.C.
8. Bozarth, M. A., and Wise, R. A. (1983): Neural substrates of opiate reinforcement. *Prog. Neuropsychopharmacol. Biol. Psychiatry,* 7:569–575.
9. Bozarth, M. A., and Wise, R. A. (1984): Anatomically distinct opiate receptor fields mediate reward and physical dependence. *Science,* 244:516–517.

10. Bozarth, M. A., and Wise, R. A. (1986): Involvement of the ventral tegmental dopamine system in opioid and psychomotor stimulant reinforcement. In: *Problems of Drug Dependence, 1985,* edited by L. S. Harris, pp. 190–196. U.S. Government Printing Office, Washington, D.C.
11. Britt, M. D., and Wise, R. A. (1983): Ventral tegmental site of opiate reward: Antagonism by a hydrophilic opiate receptor blocker. *Brain Res.,* 258:105–108.
12. Broekkamp, C. L. E., Phillips, A. G., and Cools, A. R. (1979): Facilitation of self-stimulation behavior following intracerebral microinjections of opioids into the ventral tegmental area. *Pharmacol. Biochem. Behav.,* 11:289–295.
13. Broekkamp, C. L. E., van den Bogaard, J. H., Heynen, H. J., Rops, R. H., Cools, A. R., and van Rossum, J. M. (1976): Separation of inhibiting and stimulating effects of morphine on self-stimulation behaviour by intracerebral microinjections. *Eur. J. Pharmacol.,* 36:443–446.
14. Carey, R. J. (1982): Unilateral 6-hydroxydopamine lesions of dopamine neurons produce bilateral self-stimulation deficits. *Behav. Brain Res.,* 6:101–114.
15. Carlsson, A. (1970): Amphetamine and brain catecholamines. In: *Amphetamine and Related Compounds,* edited by E. Costa and S. Garattini, pp. 289–300. Raven Press, New York.
16. Carlsson, A., Linqvist, M., and Kehr, W. (1974): Postmortem accumulation of 3-methoxytyramine in brain. *Naunyn Schmiedebergs Arch. Pharmacol.,* 284:365–372.
17. Crow, T. J. (1972): Catecholamine-containing neurons and electrical stimulation: 1. A review of some data. *Psychol. Med.,* 2:414–421.
18. Eidelberg, E. (1976): Possible actions of opiates upon synapses. *Prog. Neurobiol.,* 6:81–102.
19. Esposito, R. U., and Kornetsky, C. (1978): Opioids and rewarding brain stimulation. *Neurosci. Biobehav. Rev.,* 7:115–122.
20. Esposito, R. U., Porrino, L. J., Seeger, T. F., Crane, A. M., Everist, H. D., and Pert, A. (1984): Changes in local cerebral glucose utilization during rewarding brain stimulation. *Proc. Natl. Acad. Sci. USA,* 81:635–639.
21. Fibiger, H. C. (1978): Drugs and reinforcement mechanisms: A critical review of the catecholamine theory. *Annu. Rev. Pharmacol. Toxicol.,* 18:37–56.
22. Fibiger, H. C., and Phillips, A. G. (1979): Dopamine and the neural mechanisms of reinforcement. In: *The Neurobiology of Dopamine,* edited by A. S. Horn, B. H. C. Westerink, and J. Korf, pp. 597–615. Academic Press, New York.
23. Fouriezos, G., Hansson, P., and Wise, R. A. (1978): Neuroleptic induced attenuation of brain stimulation reward in rats. *J Comp. Physiol. Psychol.,* 92:661–671.
24. Franklin, K. B. J. (1979): Catecholamines and self-stimulation: Reward and performance deficits dissociated. *Pharmacol. Biochem. Behav.,* 10:751–760.
25. Gallistel, C. R., Gomita, Y., Yadin, E., and Campbell, K. A.: Forebrain origins and terminations of the MFB metabolically activated by rewarding stimulation or by reward-blocking doses of pimozide. *J. Neurosci.,* 5:1246–1261.
26. Gallistel, C. R., Shizgal, P., and Yeomans, J. S. (1981): A portrait of the substrate for self-stimulation. *Psychol. Rev.,* 88:228–273.
27. German, D. C., and Bowden, D. M. (1974): Catecholamine systems as the neural substrate for intracranial self-stimulation: A hypothesis. *Brain Res.,* 73:381–419.
28. Glick, S. D., and Cox, R. D. (1977): Changes in morphine self-administration after brainstem lesions in rats. *Psychopharmacology (Berlin),* 52:151–156.
29. Griffiths, R. R., and Balster, R. L. (1979): Opioids: Similarity between evaluations of subjective effects and animal self-administration results. *Clin. Pharmacol. Ther.,* 25:611–617.
30. Gysling, K., and Wang, R. Y. (1983): Morphine-induced activation of A10 dopamine neurons in the rat. *Brain Res.,* 277:119–127.
31. Hand, T. H., and Franklin, K. B. (1985): 6-OHDA lesions of the ventral tegmental area block morphine-induced but not amphetamine-induced facilitation of self-stimulation. *Brain Res.,* 328:233–241.
32. Heikkila, R. E., Orlansky, H., and Cohen, G. (1975): Studies on the distinction between uptake inhibition and release of [^{3}H]dopamine in rat brain tissue slices. *Biochem. Pharmacol.,* 24:847–852.
33. Hess, W. R. (1957): *The Functional Organization of the Diencephalon.* Grune and Stratton, New York.
34. Hoebel, B. G., Monaco, A. P., Hernandez, L., Aulisi, E. F., Stanley, B. G., and Lenard, L. (1983): Self-injection of amphetamine directly into the brain. *Psychopharmacology (Berlin),* 81:158–163.

35. Holmes, L. J., Bozarth, M. A., and Wise, R. A. (1983): Circling from intracranial morphine applied to the ventral tegmental area in rats. *Brain Res. Bull.,* 11:295–298.
36. Koob, G. F., Fray, P. J., and Iversen, S. D. (1978): Self-stimulation at the lateral hypothalamus and locus coeruleus after specific unilateral lesions of the dopamine system. *Brain Res.,* 146: 123–140.
37. Lyness, W. H., Friedle, N. M., and Moore, K. E. (1979): Destruction of dopaminergic nerve terminals in nucleus accumbens: Effect on d-amphetamine self-administration. *Pharmacol. Biochem. Behav.,* 11:553–556.
38. Matthews, R. T., and German, D. C. (1984): Electrophysiological evidence for excitation of rat ventral tegmental area dopamine neurons by morphine. *Neuroscience,* 11:617–625.
39. Murrin, L. C., and Roth, R. H. (1976): Dopaminergic neurons: Effects of electrical stimulation on dopamine biosynthesis. *Mol. Pharmacol.,* 12:463–475.
40. Olds, J. (1958): Self-stimulation of the brain. *Science,* 127:315–324.
41. Olds, J. (1977): *Drives and Reinforcements: Behavioral Studies of Hypothalamic Functions.* Raven Press, New York.
42. Olds, J., and Milner, P. M. (1954): Positive reinforcement produced by electrical stimulation of septal area and other regions of rat brain. *J Comp. Physiol. Psychol.,* 47:419–427.
43. Phillips, A. G., Mora, F., and Rolls, E. T. (1981): Intracerebral self-administration of amphetamine by rhesus monkeys. *Neurosci. Lett.,* 24:81–86.
44. Phillips, A. G., Spyraki, C., and Fibiger, H. C. (1982): Conditioned place preference with amphetamine and opiates as reward stimuli: Attenuation by haloperidol. In: *The Neural Basis of Feeding and Reward,* edited by B. G. Hoebel and D. Novin, pp. 455–464. Haer Institute, New Brunswick, Maine.
45. Reid, L. D., and Bozarth, M. A. (1978): Addictive agents and intracranial stimulation (ICS): The effects of various opioids on pressing for ICS. *Problems of Drug Dependence,* 729–741.
46. Roberts, D. C. S., Corcoran, M. E., and Fibiger, H. C. (1977): On the role of the ascending catecholaminergic systems in intravenous self-administration of cocaine. *Pharmacol. Biochem. Behav.,* 6:615–620.
47. Roberts, D. C. S., and Koob, G. F. (1982): Disruption of cocaine self-administration following 6-hydroxydopamine lesions of the ventral tegmental area in rats. *Pharmacol. Biochem. Behav.,* 17:901–904.
48. Roberts, D. C. S., Koob, G. F., Klonoff, P., and Fibiger, H. C. (1980): Extinction and recovery of cocaine self-administration following 6-hydroxydopamine lesions of the nucleus accumbens. *Pharmacol. Biochem. Behav.,* 12:781–787.
49. Roberts, D. C. S., and Zito, K. A. Interpretation of lesion effects on stimulant self-administration. In: *Methods of Assessing the Reinforcing Properties of Abused Drugs,* edited by M. A. Bozarth. (*in press*).
50. Schenk, S., Coupal, A., Williams, T., and Shizgal, P. (1981): A within-subject comparison of the effects of morphine on lateral hypothalamic and central gray self-stimulation. *Pharmacol. Biochem. Behav.,* 15:37–41.
51. Schwartz, J. C., Pollard, H., Llorens, C., Malfroy, B., Gros, C., Pradelles, P., and Dray, F. (1978): Endorphins and endorphin receptors in striatum: Relationship with dopaminergic neurons. In: *Advances in Biochemical Psychopharmacology, Vol. 18,* edited by E. Costa and M. Trabucchi, pp. 245–264. Raven Press, New York.
52. Shizgal, P., Bielajew, C., Corbett, D., Skelton, R., and Yeomans, J. (1980): Behavioral methods for inferring anatomical linkage between rewarding brain stimulation sites. *J Comp. Physiol. Psychol.,* 94:227–237.
53. Shizgal, P., Bielajew, C., and Kiss, I. (1980): Anodal hyperpolarization block technique provides evidence for rostro-caudal conduction of reward signals in the medial forebrain bundle. *Soc. Neurosci. Abstr.,* 6:422.
54. Shizgal, P., Bielajew, C., and Rompre, P.-P.: Quantitative characteristics of the directly stimulated neurons subserving self-stimulation of the medial forebrain bundle: Psychophysical inference and electrophysiological measurement. In: *Biological Determinants of Reinforcement,* edited by R. M. Church, M. L. Commons, J. R. Stellar, and A. R. Wagner. Lawrence Erlbaum Associates, Hillsdale, New Jersey (*in press*).
55. Sokoloff, L. (1981): The relationship between function and energy metabolism: Its use in the localization of functional activity in the nervous system. *Neurosci. Res. Prog. Bull.,* 19:159–210.

56. Spealman, R. D., and Goldberg, S. R. (1978): Drug self-administration by laboratory animals: Control by schedules of reinforcement. *Annu. Rev. Pharmacol. Toxicol.,* 18:313–339.
57. Stein, L. (1962): Effects and interactions of imipramine, chlorpromazine, reserpine and amphetamine on self-stimulation: Possible neurophysiological basis of depression. In: *Recent Advances in Biological Psychiatry,* edited by J. Wortis, pp. 288–308. Plenum Press, New York.
58. Ungerstedt, U. (1971): Adipsia and aphagia after 6-hydroxydopamine induced degeneration of the nigro-striatal dopamine system. *Acta Physiol. Scand.* [*Suppl.*], 367:95–122.
59. Ungerstedt, U. (1971): Striatal dopamine release after amphetamine or nerve degeneration revealed by rotational behavior. *Acta Physiol. Scand.* [*Suppl.*], 367:49–68.
60. Vaccarino, F. J., Bloom, F. E., and Koob, G. F. (1985): Blockade of nucleus accumbens opiate receptors attenuates intravenous heroin reward in the rat. *Psychopharmacology (Berlin),* 86:37–42.
61. van der Kooy, D., Mucha, R. F., O'Shaughnessy, M., and Bucenieks, P. (1982): Reinforcing effects of brain microinjections of morphine revealed by conditioned place preference. *Brain Res.,* 243:107–117.
62. van Ree, J. M., and de Wied, D. (1980): Involvement of neurohypophyseal peptides in drug-mediated adaptive responses. *Pharmacol. Biochem. Behav.,* 13(Suppl. 1):257–263.
63. Weeks, J. R., and Collins, R. J.: Screening for drug reinforcement using intravenous self-administration in the rat. In: *Methods of Assessing the Reinforcing Properties of Abused Drugs,* edited by M. A. Bozarth. (*in press*).
64. Westerink, B. H. C. (1978): Effect of centrally acting drugs on regional dopamine metabolism. In: *Advances in Biochemical Psychopharmacology, Vol. 19,* edited by P. J. Roberts, G. N. Woodruff, and L. L. Iversen, pp. 255–266. Raven Press, New York.
65. Westerink, B. H. C., and Spaan, S. J. (1982): On the significance of endogenous 3-methoxytyramine for the effects of centrally acting drugs on dopamine release in the brain. *J. Neurochem.,* 38:680–686.
66. Wise, R. A. (1978): Catecholamine theories of reward: A critical review. *Brain Res.,* 152:215–247.
67. Wise, R. A. (1983): Brain neuronal systems mediating reward processes. In: *Neurobiology of Opiate Reward Processes,* edited by J. E. Smith and J. D. Lane, pp. 405–437. Elsevier/North Holland Biomedical Press, Amsterdam.
68. Wise, R. A., Jenck, F., and Raptis, L. (1986): Morphine potentiates feeding via the opiate reinforcement mechanisms. In: *Problems of Drug Dependence, 1985,* edited by L. S. Harris, pp. 228–234. U.S. Government Printing Office, Washington, D.C.
69. Wood, P. L. (1983): Opioid regulation of CNS dopaminergic pathways: A review of methodology, receptor types, regional variations, and species differences. *Peptides,* 4:595–601.
70. Wood, P. L., Nair, N. P. V., and Bozarth, M. A. (1982): Striatal 3-methoxytyramine as an index of dopamine release: Effects of electrical stimulation. *Neurosci. Lett.,* 32:291–294.
71. Yadin, E., Guarini, V., and Gallistel, C. R. (1983): Unilaterally activated systems in rats self-stimulating at sites in the medial forebrain bundle, medial prefrontal cortex, or locus coeruleus. *Brain Res.,* 266:39–50.
72. Yeomans, J. S. (1975): Quantitative measurement of neural post-stimulation excitability with behavioral methods. *Physiol. Behav.,* 15:593–602.
73. Yokel, R. A.: Intravenous self-administration: Response rates, the effects of pharmacological challenges, and drug preferences. In: *Methods of Assessing the Reinforcing Properties of Abused Drugs,* edited by M. A. Bozarth. (*in press*).
74. Yokel, R. A., and Wise, R. A. (1975): Increased lever pressing for amphetamine after pimozide in rats: Implications for a dopamine theory of reward. *Science,* 187:547–549.
75. Yokel, R. A., and Wise, R. A. (1976): Attenuation of intravenous amphetamine reinforcement by central dopamine blockade in rats. *Psychopharmacology (Berlin),* 48:311–318.

Brain Reward Systems and Abuse, edited by
J. Engel and L. Oreland.
Raven Press, New York © 1987.

Reward Transmitters and Drugs of Abuse

Larry Stein and James D. Belluzzi

*Department of Pharmacology, College of Medicine, University of California at Irvine,
Irvine, California 92717*

To many neuroscientists, it is a contradiction to attempt to investigate the biological substrates of reward. According to these investigators, reward is merely a mentalistic concept and, as such, does not have a place in hard science. In this chapter, we shall try to explicate the concept of reward or positive reinforcement in the most concrete terms possible. We shall try to show that to identify the neuronal substrates of reward is one of the most important problems to be solved by neuroscientists interested in behavior and in the question of substance abuse.

We also shall discuss the two principal methods currently used to investigate brain reward mechanisms. We shall try to show that this methodology (despite certain shortcomings) is logically and scientifically valid and that the data generated by these methods have yielded an attractive and heuristic hypothesis concerning the anatomy and physiology of brain reward systems. Then we shall discuss drugs of abuse—drugs such as heroin and cocaine—which we shall describe as pharmacological rewards. We shall argue, consistently with the theme of this volume, that natural rewards and pharmacological rewards act on the brain's reinforcement mechanism in essentially similar ways to regulate behavior. Indeed, we shall argue that natural rewards and addictive drugs may activate the same brain cells or brain receptors to initiate the reward process. Finally, we shall describe our recent work at the cellular level, which also suggests similarities in the mechanisms of reward and drug abuse.

POSITIVE REINFORCEMENT: CONTROL BY CONSEQUENCES

The concept of reward or positive reinforcement, as defined in this chapter, does not refer to subjective feelings of pleasure and is not related to hedonic valuation. The concept refers exclusively to the question of how stimuli control behavior. According to Skinner (14), environmental stimuli can control behavior in two fundamentally different ways (Fig. 1). First, there is a respondent or reflex-like process (stimulus–response), in which the controlling environmental stimulus precedes and elicits the response. Most neuroscientists are comfortable with the concept of respondent control, since it is similar or identical to the traditional

Control by Antecedents

Reflexes

S--R

FIG. 1. Scheme of Skinner (14) showing that environmental stimuli can control behavior in either of two ways: respondent (control by antecedents) or operant (control by consequences). S, stimulus; R, response.

Control by Consequences

Reinforced Behaviors

R--S

reflex of classic physiology and since the underlying brain organization has been extensively explored. The second kind of control process (response–stimulus), which Skinner terms "operant," is more troublesome. In the operant case, the controlling environmental stimulus (reward object) follows the response and increases its subsequent probability. Why is operant control, or control by consequences, so troublesome to many neuroscientists? There are at least three reasons.

Response Initiation

According to Skinner (14), operant responses are emitted and not elicited. If so, how does the response get started in the absence of an eliciting stimulus? The current view of a spontaneously active brain (versus the older view of a passive one) makes Skinner's idea of spontaneous response emission more acceptable than previously.

Control by Consequences

Control by consequences seems to violate conventional ideas of causality. How can a rewarding stimulus influence a response that has already been completed? As Skinner (16) has argued, the selection of successful responses by reinforcing stimuli has the same logical status as the natural selection of successful structures and functions in evolutionary biology. Both are examples of selection by consequences—a causal mode found only in living things—in contrast to the causal mode common in physical science (i.e., causality by an initiating agent).

Unconventional Circuitry

When the controlling stimulus precedes the response, as in the conventional reflex arc, information flow in the brain is afferent to efferent; on the other hand,

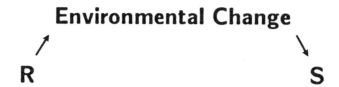

FIG. 2. The neuronal substrate of reinforced responses (R) is not directly connected to and does not directly activate the neuronal substrate of goal-detecting sensory systems (S). Rather, the correct response causes an environmental change, which in turn activates the goal-detecting sensory system.

when the controlling stimulus follows the response, as in the case of operant behavior, the underlying brain organization seems to require an unconventional circuitry in which efferents are activated before afferents. However, the mechanisms for reinforced behavior do not require circuits that directly link efferent to afferent elements. This is because reinforced responses do not directly activate goal-detecting afferent systems. Rather, the correct response operates on the environment to produce the goal object, and it is this environmental change that activates the goal-detecting systems (Fig. 2). Thus, although the reinforcement mechanism does not require efferent-to-afferent circuitry, it must recognize and be activated by efferent–afferent contingencies; i.e., it must cause behavioral reinforcement only when the neuronal substrates of the correct response and goal object, in that order, are activated sequentially.

The problem of characterizing the brain reinforcement mechanism has two main parts. The first is to identify the neurons or neuronal substrate that performs the reinforcing function. We assume this substrate is neurochemically specialized and will call these specialized neurons "reward neurons." The second part of the brain reinforcement problem is to identify the neuronal substrate that is modified by the reinforcement process (we will call these the "target" neurons).

REWARD NEURONS

The idea that reinforcing functions are specialized neurochemically has guided research in this field for more than 25 years. The alternative possibility that these functions are not neurochemically specialized has not been disproved, but this view has not proved heuristic. The hypothesis (18) that certain catecholamine and endorphin brain cells may serve as reinforcing neurons is supported by evidence from brain self-stimulation and drug self-administration experiments. In the self-stimulation experiments, animals work to deliver electrical stimulation to their own brains through permanently indwelling electrodes (Fig. 3). In the absence of other sources of reward, the reinforcement for self-stimulation behavior must arise from the neuronal activity that is excited by the electrical stimulus. Although such centrally elicited reinforcement could be an artifact, it more plausibly represents a process based on natural physiology. If so, it would be logical to assume that some of the neurons under the electrode tip actually are the

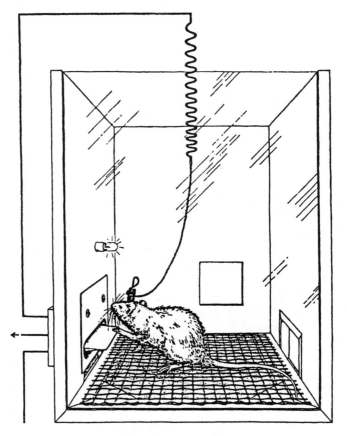

FIG. 3. Diagram of the self-stimulation circuit of Olds and Milner (12). When the rat presses the lever it triggers a rewarding electric stimulus to its brain.

reward neurons that mediate the effects of natural reinforcers or at least are neurons that directly excite them.

High self-stimulation rates are observed when electrodes are implanted in regions containing catecholamine or endorphin cell bodies or pathways (2,4,12,17). In particular, self-stimulation tightly overlaps the distribution of dopamine cells in the ventral tegmentum and substantia nigra. Self-stimulation closely follows the anteriorly projecting dopamine fibers through the hypothalamus, but it correlates somewhat less closely with the dopamine terminal fields in the forebrain. The involvement of norepinephrine neurons in self-stimulation is still a matter of controversy. Although many laboratories report self-stimulation from sites in the vicinity of the locus ceruleus, it has not been possible to establish convincingly that the noradrenergic neurons that make up this nucleus are responsible for the reinforcing effect (8). Preliminary mapping of endorphin sites for self-stimulation is consistent with the idea that certain endorphin (possibly, enkephalin and β-endorphin) neurons are involved in self-stimulation (2,19), but these studies are still in a very early stage. The catecholamine–endorphin reinforcement hypothesis also is supported by pharmacological experiments. Antagonists of dopamine and endorphins, such as haloperidol and naloxone, respectively, should block chemical transmission of reinforcement messages. In support of the model, there are many reports that these drugs selectively block self-stimulation (2,6,10).

In self-administration experiments, behavior is reinforced by central or systemic injections of neurotransmitters or drugs. Of thousands of chemical substances available, animals and humans avidly self-administer only a few. These self-administered substances may properly be termed pharmacological rewards, and it is interesting to ask why these chemicals are selectively associated with behavioral reinforcement. It may be no coincidence that most powerful pharmacological rewards have the ability to mimic or release the hypothesized natural reinforcement transmitters. Thus, many catecholamine and endorphin receptor activators are known to support self-administration behavior. In particular, the naturally occurring opioid peptides leu- and met-enkephalin and β-endorphin and certain degradation-resistant analogs function as positive reinforcers (2,9,13). Similarly, dopamine receptor agonists such as apomorphine and piribedil and the norepinephrine agonist clonidine are self-administered (1,22). The patterns of self-administration of these receptor agonists often resemble the patterns observed when highly addictive stimulant drugs (e.g., cocaine and amphetamine) or opiate drugs (e.g., morphine and heroin) are self-administered (1). The pharmacology of stimulant and opiate drugs closely resembles that of natural catecholamines or endorphins. Hence, it is reasonable to suppose that addiction to stimulant or opiate drugs may largely depend on their ability to activate or to enhance the activity of natural catecholamine or endorphin reinforcement systems, respectively. Finally, catecholamine and endorphin antagonists, such as chlorpromazine and naloxone, not only appropriately block the reinforcing effects of agents that activate catecholamine or endorphin receptors but also appropriately block the reinforcing effects of stimulant and opiate drugs.

The self-administration method also has been used in attempts to identify the sites of action of stimulants and opiates. In some studies, animals are trained to self-inject cocaine and morphine directly into the brain in an attempt to find preferred sites for reinforcing effects. In other studies, catecholamine or endorphin antagonists are injected into different brain regions during intravenous self-administration of drugs of abuse. Although preliminary data suggest that important sites of action for both stimulant and opiate drugs are concentrated in the nucleus

TABLE 1. *Strengths and weaknesses of self-stimulation and self-administration*

	Strength	Weakness
Self-administration	Chemical purity	Unnatural receptor activation
Self-stimulation	Natural receptor activation	Neurotransmitter heterogeneity

TABLE 2. *Hypotheses relating brain reinforcement systems and drug abuse*

Agents such as heroin and cocaine are abused because the drugs themselves are powerful reinforcers

Reinforcement processes are regulated by specialized systems of dopamine and endorphin neurons

The rewarding properties of cocaine-like and heroin-like drugs derive from the pharmacological similarities between these agents and the dopamine and endorphin reinforcement systems, respectively

The same biological process underlies addiction at three levels—cells, animals, and humans

accumbens, it is almost certain that the reinforcing action of the drugs is more widely distributed.

Although these anatomical and pharmacological findings seem consistent with the idea that reinforcing functions are performed by specialized systems of catecholamine and endorphin neurons, important problems remain. Administration of pure substances in the self-administration experiments strictly controls the chemical nature of the reinforcing injection, but because the distribution of injected transmitters to active sites cannot exactly duplicate that of naturally released transmitters, the ensuing pattern of receptor activation could be artifactual or misleading (Table 1). On the other hand, while electrical activation of transmitter pathways during self-stimulation presumably releases the reinforcing chemical messenger in a relatively natural distribution at appropriate postsynaptic sites, the electrical stimulus also must cause the simultaneous release of many irrelevant transmitters and neurohormones, including some that are still unknown. Thus, in the case of self-stimulation, identification of which cells and which transmitters are relevant to the reinforcement process is largely a matter of inference. Solutions may be based on mapping studies, which demonstrate self-stimulation in anatomically coherent systems, and on pharmacological studies, which implicate specific neurotransmitters. However, the anatomical mapping data from most self-stimulation experiments are insufficiently detailed. At the same time, many of the pharmacological reports can be criticized because it is difficult to distinguish specific drug effects on reinforcement from nonspecific effects on performance. Self-administration studies generally provide a stronger line of evidence for catecholamine–endorphin involvement in reinforcement processes, but self-administration of the hypothesized natural reinforcing transmitters—dopamine and norepinephrine—has not been reported. The assumptions relating the catecholamine–endorphin reward hypothesis to the present theory of substance abuse are summarized in Table 2.

CELLULAR ASPECTS OF REWARD AND ABUSE

As noted above, little consideration or experimental effort has been devoted to the identification of the substrate that is modified by the reinforcement process, i.e., the neuronal targets of the reinforcing neurons. Since it is behavior that is reinforced, it is plausible to assume that neuronal substrates of behavior are major targets. A behavioral response obviously reflects the activity of many neurons. Is it the integrated activity of these neurons that is reinforced; that is, is reinforcement exerted at the level of neuronal circuits or cell assemblies? Or is it the individual activities of the relevant neurons that is reinforced; that is, is reinforcement exerted at the cellular level? It is commonly believed that the reinforcement of behavior is paralleled at the neuronal level by the strengthening or reorganization of complex neuronal circuits. Unfortunately, no such circuit or cell assembly for any reinforced behavior has yet been identified. Where in the rat's brain, for example, would one find the circuit for a lever-press response? And how would one measure the changes in circuitry that are induced when lever-pressing is reinforced? These anatomical and physiological considerations, as well as difficulties at the behavioral level associated with response definition, have led some scientists to ask whether it really is correct to say that the whole response is the functional unit for reinforcement. According to Skinner (15), a more useful conceptual scheme assumes that all responses are made up of elements and that it is these elements or "behavioral atoms," and not whole responses, that are the units strengthened by reinforcement. If so and if atoms of behavior can be represented by the activity of individual neurons, then it could be argued that it is the behavior not of neuronal circuits but of individual neurons that is directly modified by reinforcing signals (7). This idea can be tested by attempting to demonstrate that the activity of isolated brain cells can be reinforced by local applications of appropriate transmitters or drugs.

OPERANT CONDITIONING OF INDIVIDUAL NEURONS

Olds (11) was the first to report apparent evidence for the operant conditioning of single neurons. In these experiments, rats with implanted microelectrodes received food or rewarding brain stimulation contingent on appropriate bursts of single-unit activity. Firing rates were increased in a number of cases, suggesting reinforcement of the single-unit response. Unfortunately, it is not clear whether it was the behavior of the individual neuron that was being reinforced or whether some more complex response or movement, of which the neuron's activity was a part, was actually being reinforced. In some of Olds' tests, a restriction system was used to limit movement: electronic detectors were discharged by most movements, and these precluded reinforcement. Although operant conditioning was still obtained under these conditions, one cannot rule out the possible reinforcement of behaviors involving undetected movements, such as postural adjustments or attentional responses. Like other investigators who have attempted to demonstrate operant conditioning of single-unit activity (5,21), Olds recognized that, if a reinforcing stimulus is delivered to a behaving animal, it is impossible to separate the reinforcement of single units from the reinforcement of more complex responses.

Our solutions to this problem are (a) to use a greatly reduced experimental preparation—the brain slice—and (b) to deliver the reinforcing stimulus only to the neuron being conditioned. But what is effective reinforcement for a single neuron in a brain slice? According to the catecholamine–endorphin theory, reinforcement signals normally are delivered to their neuronal targets by the release of catecholamines or endorphins. If so, it might be possible to duplicate these natural signals of reinforcement by the direct application of the transmitters to appropriate neurons. In such experiments, catecholamines or endorphins would be applied via micropipettes to individual units in various regions of the brain following particular rates or patterns of activity. These rates or patterns should be strengthened only by contingent application of the transmitters and not by noncontingent application.

The experimental protocol is shown in Fig. 4 (3,20). A somewhat arbitrary decision was made in choosing which aspect of unit activity to reinforce. Since firing rates are likely to be an important vehicle for information transmission, peak rates should have high information value and might be amenable to conditioning. Thus, in these experiments, a half-second period of relatively rapid activity was defined as the neuronal response to be reinforced (Fig. 5). These neuronal responses or "bursts" were individually determined for each unit studied. Prior to the start of conditioning, 500 successive half-second samples of

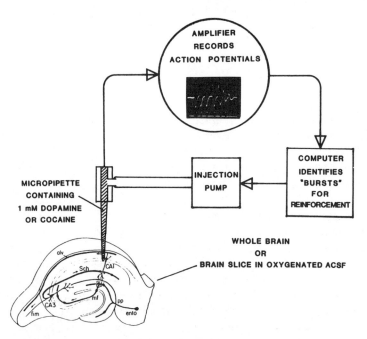

FIG. 4. Protocol for operant conditioning of individual brain cells. A burst of firing of a hippocampal pyramidal cell in area CA1 activates a pressure injection pump which puffs a microinjection of dopamine or cocaine in the close vicinity of the active cell.

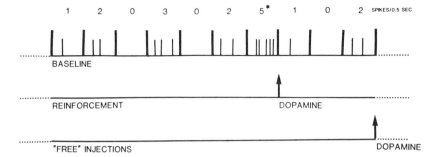

FIG. 5. Diagram of procedure for defining and reinforcing neuronal responses. Spike activity is counted and summed arbitrarily in bins of 0.5-sec duration. Prior to experiment proper, baseline recordings are made for each neuron under investigation to determine a suitable criterion response for later reinforcement. Bins that contain *n* or more spikes are followed by reinforcement, where *n* is that number of spikes in a bin that is equalled or exceeded in approximately 5% of all bins sampled. *Criterion response.

neuronal activity were recorded, and a frequency distribution of the number of spikes per sample was compiled. A "burst" was defined as that spike number equalled or exceeded in only 1 to 8% of the samples.

The basic operant conditioning method involved six stages:

(a) Baseline. The number of bursts in the absence of reinforcement (operant level) was determined during a baseline period of approximately 10 min.

(b) Operant conditioning. Each burst was followed by an injection of the reinforcing solution. If conditioning failed to occur after 5 min, the duration of the injection (and hence the dose) was increased until evidence of conditioning was obtained or until direct pharmacological or mechanical effects interfered with recording.

(c) Extinction. Reinforcement was terminated, and recording continued until the baseline was recovered.

(d) Matched free injections. Noncontingent injections of the reinforcing solution were made at regular intervals to determine direct pharmacological effects on rates of firing and probability of bursts. The pattern and number of free injections were matched to the pattern and number of reinforcing injections in the preceding phase of operant conditioning. The presentation of programmed free injections was delayed for 3 sec after the occurrence of bursts to minimize their adventitious reinforcement.

(e) Washout. A second baseline period without injections was given in order to allow residual effects of the noncontingent drug administrations to be dissipated.

(f) Reacquisition. A second period of reinforcement was scheduled, whenever possible, in order to compare rates of original acquisition and reacquisition.

Results from a positive experiment using dopamine as the reinforcing solution are shown for a hippocampal unit in Fig. 6. The frequency of bursts and overall

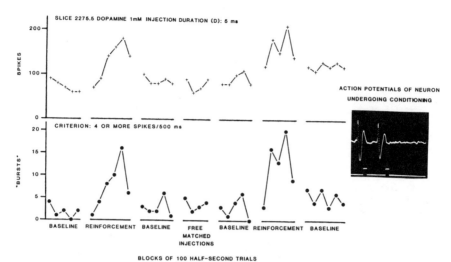

FIG. 6. Operant conditioning of the activity of a CA1 pyramidal cell in a slice of dorsal hippocampus with local injections of dopamine as reinforcement. The activity of the unit throughout seven phases of a complete experiment is shown. Each point shows the number of bursts (*lower graph*) and the total number of spikes (*upper graph*) in successive blocks of 100 half-second samples or trials. Prior to the first baseline phase, a burst criterion of 4 or more spikes/half-sec sample was selected. This criterion gave a burst rate for this unit that never exceeded 4% in the initial baseline period. In the reinforcement phase, dopamine HCl (1 mM in 165 mM saline) was applied for 5 msec immediately after each burst. Following a second baseline period, the same dopamine injections were delivered independently of the unit's behavior as a control for possible stimulant effects. The number of injections was matched to that earned during the last four periods of the reinforcement phase. Burst and overall spike rates were increased by the contingent dopamine injections during the reinforcement phase but were not increased when the same injections were administered noncontingently in the free matched injection phase. **Inset.** *Upper trace:* Photograph of digital oscilloscope display of two action potentials from the unit undergoing conditioning. *Lower trace:* 1-msec time markers.

firing rates were rapidly increased after approximately 10 dopamine reinforcements in two separate phases of operant conditioning (marked "reinforcement" in Fig. 6). The same dopamine injections administered noncontingently ("free matched injections") failed to increase either burst frequency or overall firing rate. It may also be noted that extinction occurred rapidly after both instances of operant conditioning. A second experiment, in which cocaine was used to reinforce neuronal activity, is summarized in Fig. 7. In this experiment, free injections of cocaine were given both before and after the reinforcement phase. The initial phase of free injections, delivered at a rate of 5 injections/min, had no apparent effect on neuronal activity. However, reinforcing applications of cocaine produced sharp increases in bursts and overall firing rate. This increased firing rate was sustained for several minutes of extinction (third "baseline" period) after which they rapidly declined. Free cocaine injections, matched in frequency to the peak rate obtained in the preceding reinforcement phase, again had a negligible effect on the number of bursts or the overall firing rate. In a second phase of reinforcement ("reinf"), contingent injections of cocaine again increased

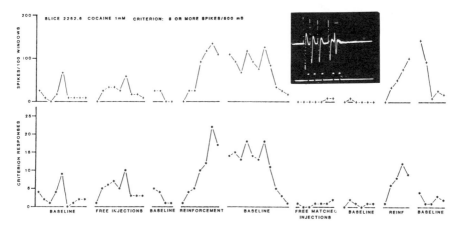

FIG. 7. Operant conditioning of a pyramidal neuron in a dorsal hippocampal slice using local injections of cocaine as reinforcement. For details, see text and Fig. 6. Free, noncontingent injections phase; reinf., reinforcement phase.

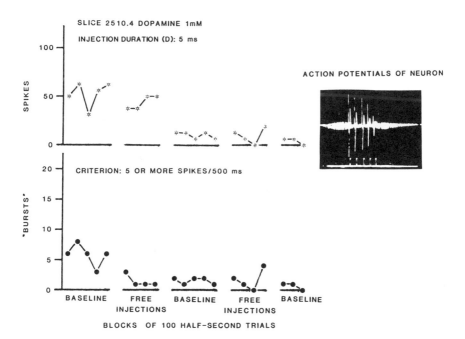

FIG. 8. Control experiment with dopamine administered noncontingently to a pyramidal neuron in hippocampal slice. For details, see text and Fig. 6.

the frequency of bursts and the overall firing rate but not to the level observed in the first reinforcement phase. In control experiments, dopamine was administered noncontingently throughout the experiment, or saline was substituted for dopamine (Figs. 8 and 9, respectively). In neither case was the burst frequency or overall firing rate increased.

A summary of eight positive dopamine experiments is shown in Fig. 10. Plotted here are the means of the peak rates obtained in each phase of the experiment for each neuron. Highly significant increases were obtained in each of the reinforcement periods when compared either to baseline control periods or to periods ("matched") during which the same number of dopamine injections was presented independently of neuronal bursting. A similar summary of the positive cocaine experiments is shown in Fig. 11.

Finally, a general summary of experiments with a number of different transmitters and drugs is presented in Table 3. Excluded are many experiments in which suitable action potentials could not be obtained or held, or in which artifacts, such as drug overdoses or clogging of the micropipette, caused experiments to be abandoned. In the columns labeled "Results," the designations are defined as follows: +, conditioning-like changes (increased probability of bursts following reinforcement) plus noncontingent controls; ?, conditioning-like changes but no controls; and —, no evidence of conditioning. The table thus

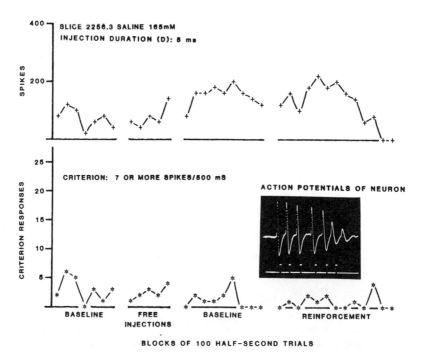

FIG. 9. Saline control experiment. Failure to obtain evidence of operant conditioning of a pyramidal neuron in dorsal hippocampal slice with local injections of saline as reinforcement. For details, see text and Fig. 6.

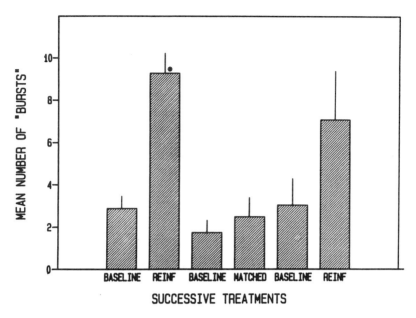

FIG. 10. Summary of positive dopamine experiments. $N = 8$; vertical lines represent SEMs. *$p < 0.05$.

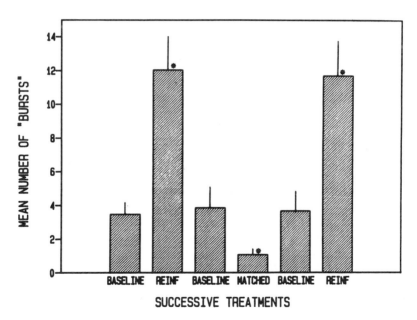

FIG. 11. Summary of positive cocaine experiments. $N = 11$, vertical lines represent SEMs. *$p < 0.05$.

TABLE 3. *Summary of hippocampal brain-slice experiments*

Drug	Dose (mM)	No. of experiments	Results[a]		
			+	?	—
Cocaine	1	48	11	12	25
Cocaine (free)	1	13	0	0	13
Dopamine	1	17	9	2	6
Dopamine (free)	1	12	0	1	11
Norepinephrine	1	4	1	1	2
Acetylcholine	1	6	1	1	4
Serotonin	1	3	0	0	3
GABA	1	4	0	0	4
Amphetamine	1	3	0	2	1
Imipramine	1	2	0	0	2
Ethanol	1	3	0	0	3
Saline	165	5	0	0	5

[a] Columns are defined as follows: +, conditioning-like changes (increased probability of bursts following reinforcement) plus noncontingent controls; ?, conditioning-like changes, but no controls; —, no evidence of conditioning.

indicates that 9 of the 17 completed dopamine experiments were positive and contained noncontingent controls. In the cocaine experiments, the success rate was substantially lower than in the dopamine experiments. We do not know the explanation but speculate that cocaine, which acts via dopamine, may require a physiologically active dopamine system to exert its full reinforcing effect. Since the dopamine axons are severed in the hippocampal-slice preparation, it is conceivable that their responsivity to cocaine is reduced. With only two exceptions, positive experiments were not obtained in our preliminary tests (at a single dose level) with other agents.

CONCLUSIONS

Cellular applications of dopamine or cocaine to spontaneously active pyramidal cells in slices of rat hippocampus had opposite effects on subsequent firing rates depending on the activity pattern of the neuron at the time of administration. When the neuron had been firing rapidly just before the injection, the firing rate was increased. However, when the neuron had been firing slowly or was silent just before the injection, the firing rate was unaffected or decreased. In other words, the action of locally applied dopamine or cocaine on hippocampal cells was activity-related in a way that formally resembles the action of conventional reinforcers on behavior. A food pellet delivered after a lever-press response increases lever-pressing, whereas the same pellet delivered independently of the behavior has no effect or may even suppress lever-pressing. These observations, therefore, are consistent with the possibility that individual neurons may be operantly conditioned by direct cellular applications of reinforcing transmitters or drugs. If so and since it is unlikely that a brain cell would display a gratuitous capacity for operant conditioning, it is possible to speculate that the individual neuron may be an important organizational unit in the brain for positive reinforcement and, by extrapolation, for drug abuse.

ACKNOWLEDGMENTS

This work was supported by AFOSR grant 84-0325. We thank Charlotte Hoffmann and Eve Chan for expert technical assistance.

REFERENCES

1. Baxter, B. L., Gluckman, M. I., Stein, L., and Scerni, R. A. (1974): Self-injection of apomorphine in the rat: Positive reinforcement by a dopamine receptor stimulant. *Pharmacol. Biochem. Behav.*, 2:387–391.
2. Belluzzi, J. D., and Stein, L. (1977): Enkephalin may mediate euphoria and drive-reduction reward. *Nature*, 266:556–558.
3. Belluzzi, J. D., and Stein, L. (1983): Operant conditioning: Cellular or systems property? *Society for Neuroscience Abstracts*, 9:478.
4. Crow, T. J. (1972): A map of the rat mesencephalon for electrical stimulation. *Brain Res.*, 36: 265–273.
5. Fetz, E. E. (1969): Operant conditioning of cortical unit activity. *Science*, 163:955–958.
6. Holtzman, S. G. (1976): Comparison of the effects of morphine, pentazocine, cyclazocine and amphetamine on intracranial self-stimulation in the rat. *Psychopharmacology (Berlin)*, 46:223–227.
7. Klopf, A. H. (1982): *The Hedonistic Neuron: A Theory of Memory, Learning, and Intelligence.* Hemisphere Press, Washington, D.C.
8. Loughlin, S. E., Belluzzi, J. D., Leslie, F. M., and Stein, L. (1983): Self-stimulation in the region of locus coeruleus: Opioid or catecholaminergic mechanisms? *Society for Neuroscience Abstracts*, 9:277.
9. Mello, N. K., and Mendelson, J. H. (1979): Self-administration of an enkephalin analog by rhesus monkey. *Pharmacol. Biochem. Behav.*, 9:579–586.
10. Olds, J. (1962): Hypothalamic substrates of reward. *Physiol. Rev.*, 42:554–604.
11. Olds, J. (1965): Operant conditioning of single unit responses. *Excerpta Medica International Congress Series*, No. 87, 372–380.
12. Olds, J., and Milner, P. M. (1954): Positive reinforcement produced by electrical stimulation of septal area and other regions of rat brain. *Journal of Comparative and Physiological Psychology*, 47:419–427.
13. Olds, M. E., and Williams, K. N. (1980): Self-administration of D-Ala[2]-Met-enkephalinamide at hypothalamic self-stimulation sites. *Brain Res.*, 194:155–170.
14. Skinner, B. F. (1938): *The Behavior of Organisms: An Experimental Analysis.* Appleton-Century-Crofts, New York.
15. Skinner, B. F. (1953): *Science and Human Behavior.* The Free Press, New York.
16. Skinner, B. F. (1981): Selection by consequences. *Science*, 213:501–504.
17. Stein, L. (1964): Self-stimulation of the brain and central stimulant action of amphetamine. *Fed. Proc.*, 23:836–850.
18. Stein, L. (1978): Reward transmitters: Catecholamines and opioid peptides. In: *Psychopharmacology: A Generation of Progress*, edited by M. A. Lipton, A. DiMascio, and K. F. Killam, pp. 569–581. Raven Press, New York.
19. Stein, L., and Belluzzi, J. D. (1979): Brain endorphins: Possible role in reward and memory formation. *Fed. Proc.*, 38:2468–2472.
20. Stein, L., and Belluzzi, J. D. (1985): Operant conditioning of hippocampal neurons: Chlorpromazine blocks reinforcing actions of dopamine. *Society for Neuroscience Abstracts*, 11:873.
21. Wyler, A. R., and Robbins, C. A. (1980): Operant control of precentral neurons: The role of audio and visual feedback. *Exp. Neurol.*, 70:200–203.
22. Yokel, R. A., and Wise, R. A. (1976): Attenuation of intravenous amphetamine reinforcement by central dopamine blockade in rats. *Psychopharmacology (Berlin)*, 48:311–318.

Brain Reward Systems and Abuse, edited by
J. Engel and L. Oreland.
Raven Press, New York © 1987.

Positive Reinforcement Properties of Drugs: Search for Neural Substrates

George F. Koob, Franco Vaccarino, Marianne Amalric, and
Floyd E. Bloom

*Division of Preclinical Neuroscience and Endocrinology, Scripps Clinic and Research
Foundation, La Jolla, California 92037*

Drugs can function both as discriminative stimuli and consequence events in establishing and controlling operant behavior. The general thesis of operant conditioning is that behavior that operates upon the environment is controlled by its consequences. Those consequences that strengthen behavior are called "reinforcers" (an event that increases the probability of a response). A drug serving as controlling consequence for the operant behavior leading to its administration is therefore defined as a "reinforcer."

The experimental analysis of the biological and environmental variables that modify a drug's reinforcing efficacy—i.e., the extent to which a drug is self-administered—has obvious implications for research on problems of human drug-seeking behavior and dependence. Humans have self-administered chemical substances since before recorded history, and such self-administration in excessive or inappropriate amounts has been termed "drug abuse" or even "drug addiction."

DRUGS AS REINFORCERS

Drugs are readily self-administered by animals (39), and there are now several extensive reviews documenting the extent to which drugs can act as reinforcers and how drugs as reinforcers act similarly to other consequent events (26,33). The validity of a rat model of intravenous self-administration has been explored by various investigators, and over the last 23 years at least 29 psychoactive drugs have been shown to support intravenous self-administration (Table 1). Further, in a recent study (7) of the drugs self-administered by primates, only ethanol failed to produce reliable intravenous self-administration in rats. Other drugs not readily self-administered in rats include cyclazocine, naloxone, caffeine, diazepam, phenobarbital, imipramine, chlorpromazine, haloperidol, ketamine, netopam, and phenytoin (7). Cyclazocine, naloxone, caffeine, imipramine, chlorpromazine, and haloperidol also are inactive in primates (7). These results

TABLE 1. *Drugs self-administered*
intravenously by rats

cocaine[c]	
d-amphetamine[g]	
l-amphetamine[g]	nalbuphine[c]
methamphetamine[c]	nalorphine[c]
methylphenidate[c]	ethylketazocine[c]
apomorphine[a]	butorphanol[c]
nicotine[c]	pentazocine[c]
heroin[e]	flurazepam[c]
morphine[c]	methohexital[c]
methadone[b]	pentobarbital[c]
codeine[c]	amobarbital[d]
l-α-acetylmethadol[h]	ethanol[f]
dihydromorphine[b]	
meperidine[c]	phencyclidine[c]
propoxyphene[c]	procaine[c]
etonitazene[c]	ACTH[e]

[a] Baxter et al. (1976): *Pharmacol. Biochem. Behav.*, 4:611–612.

[b] Collins and Weeks (1965): *N. S. Arch. Exp. Path. Pharmak.*, 249:509–514.

[c] Collins et al. (1984): *Psychopharmacology (Berlin)*, 82:6–13.

[d] Jouhaneau-Bowers et al. (1979): *Pharmacol. Biochem. Behav.*, 10:325-328.

[e] Koob et al. (1984): *J. Pharmacol. Exp. Ther.*, 229:481–486.

[f] Sinden et al. (1982): *Pharmacol. Biochem. Behav.*, 16:181–183.

[g] Yokel and Pickens (1973): *J. Pharmacol. Exp. Ther.*, 187:27–33.

[h] Young et al. (1978): *Drug Alcohol Depend*, 3:273–279.

support the hypothesis that drug self-administration in animals may be a reliable predictor of abuse liability in humans, a thesis previously suggested for animal studies based largely on primate studies (12).

There are a number of major advantages of drug self-administration to study the reinforcing properties. First, operationally, the self-administration of a drug by an animal is a direct measure of the reinforcing properties of the drug. The drug increases the probability of a response and thus acts as a reinforcer. This construct allows the use of classic operant techniques for the measures of the motivational value of a drug, allows the measure of relative reinforcement value of drugs, and allows, while controlling for nonspecificity of action, for the assessment of treatment effects.

A common simple assessment of drug self-administration employs a continuous reinforcement schedule or fixed ratio schedules of reinforcement. Here, nondependent rats typically maintain a stable amount of drug intake that varies inversely with drug dose (Fig. 1). Minimal increases in the response requirements

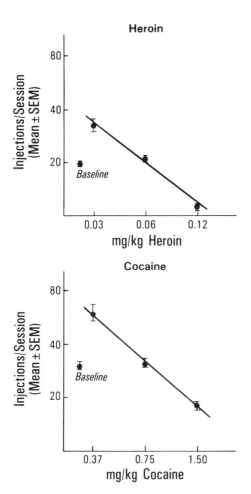

FIG. 1. Dose-response relationships for cocaine and heroin self-administration in rats. Rats were allowed daily 3-hr access to cocaine (*bottom*) (0.75 mg/kg/injection) or heroin (*top*) (0.06 mg/kg/injection) on a continuous reinforcement schedule. After baseline stable responding (±20% mean for 3 days) was established, rats were subjected to a doubling of the dose, followed by a return to baseline, followed by a halving of the dose on 3 successive test days. Results are expressed as mean ± SEM; $N = 4$.

have little effect on drug intake, but response rates increase to accommodate the ratio requirements (27).

For measures of relative reinforcement of drugs or comparisons of drugs to other reinforcers, protocols such as the progressive ratio schedule may be useful. In a progressive ratio schedule, the ratio requirement for obtaining an intravenous injection of drugs is systemically increased until the animal ceases to respond. This pause in responding is defined as the breaking point and has been used to successfully discriminate among drugs (2,13,14,27–29,43).

A second advantage of drug self-administration is that the clear dose-effect functions can be obtained even in continuous reinforcement situations, and these dose-effect functions lend themselves to pharmacological antagonism (Fig. 2). Here a competitive antagonism results in a shift of the dose-effect function to the right, which at certain doses is reflected in an actual increase in responding

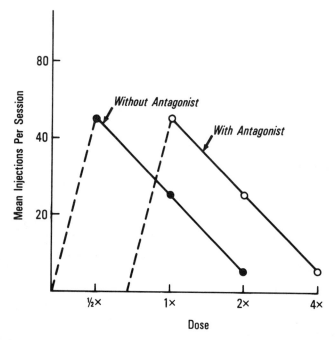

FIG. 2. Hypothetical model of the effects of a pharmacological antagonist on the dose-response function with self-administration. Note the shift of the dose-response function to the right. With this model a decrease in reinforcement value is reflected in an increase in the number of drug injections self-administered.

for the drug. This allows some degree of control for nonspecificity of action; i.e., a simple decrease in behavior due to a putative competitive antagonism may instead only reflect an inability to respond.

The third advantage of self-administration for the study of drug reinforcement is that this procedure can be used to study the biological site of action of drugs. All the techniques described above can be used to evaluate treatment effects from which inferences about function can be derived. Systemic and local intra-cerebral injections of pharmacological antagonists and neurochemically specific neurotoxins can be combined with these behavioral procedures to define the site and mechanism of action for the reinforcing properties of drugs.

BIOLOGICAL SITES FOR DRUG REINFORCEMENT

Opiates

In opiate self administration, rats who are not physically dependent maintain a relatively stable level of drug intake over time, with very regular interinjection intervals, particularly with short daily sessions (approximately 3 hr) (9,17). In response to changes in this injection dose, animals typically show an inverse relationship between dose and number of injections per session; e.g., low doses produce a higher number of self-injections than higher doses (Fig. 1). More important for the present context is the nature of the change in behavior following treatment with a pharmacological antagonist. Treatment with the opiate receptor antagonist produces an increase in the number of self-injections of morphine (9,11,40). This increase is generally considered to reflect a competitive functional interaction; the rat presumably increases its drug self-administration to compensate for the decreased effectiveness of morphine as a reinforcer in the presence of partial receptor occupancy by the antagonist. Consequently, an increase in self-administration resulting from administration of an opiate antagonist is qualitatively similar to the effects of decreasing the dose of drug per injection. A hypothetical description of this relationship is shown in Fig. 2.

In humans, opiate injection is accompanied by an intense sensation likened in quality to sexual orgasm. Known as the "rush," this sensation lasts for approximately 45 sec and is generally thought to be one of the motivating factors involved in opiate use (15). However, it is not clear that this rush is mediated by direct drug action in the CNS, since it is well established that interoceptive autonomic stimuli have an important role in the maintenance of heroin consumption in humans (20).

To test whether the reinforcing properties of opiate arise directly from activation of opiate receptors in the CNS or from opiate receptors localized in the periphery, we examined the potency and efficacy of naloxone and naltrexone with their quaternary derivatives in antagonizing the reinforcing properties of heroin. The quaternary derivatives of naloxone and naltrexone were chosen because of their potentially selective antagonist action, which excludes them from penetrating through the blood-brain barrier. As a result they can antagonize opiate effects on peripheral opiate receptors, as inferred from their ability to antagonize morphine effects on gastrointestinal transit, but do not antagonize central opiate actions on pain (36). Recent studies have confirmed conditionally the peripheral selectivity of these compounds (3).

In rats self-administering heroin (0.06 mg/kg/injection in daily 3-hr sessions), low doses (0.05 to 0.2 mg/kg) of naloxone and naltrexone produced dose-dependent increases in self-administration; at higher doses (10 to 30 mg/kg) these drugs produced transient decreases in heroin self-administration followed by recovery (9,17). The quaternary derivatives injected systemically were ineffective as antagonists of heroin self-administration in doses 200 times greater than the effective antagonist dose of naloxone or naltrexone (17) (Fig. 3). These results support the hypothesis that the acute reinforcing properties of intravenous opiates associated with the sensation of the rush involve opiate receptors located within the CNS and do not involve peripheral opiate receptors (17). The present results also are unlikely to be explained simply on the basis of differential binding potency of the antagonists to opiate receptors. Naloxone is only about 10 times more potent than methylnaloxone in displacing tritiated [D-ALA-2-Me-phe 4-Glyol 5]enkephalin (DAGO) binding (G. F. Koob, L. Randolph, and C. Chavkin, *unpublished results*, 1985).

Identification of a possible CNS site of action for the reinforcing properties of

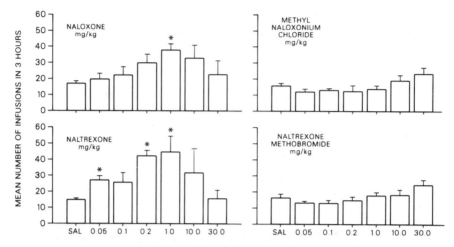

FIG. 3. Effects of naloxone, methylnaloxonium chloride, naltrexone, and naltrexone methobromide on responding over the total 3-hr test session for rats self-administering heroin. Data are expressed as mean ± SEM of the total infusions for 3 hr. *Asterisks* indicate that the treatment dose was reliably different from the saline (SAL) pretreatment condition; $p < 0.05$, paired t-test. Note that the SAL group represents mean ± SEM of all the SAL observations (which is equal to the number of different rats used in each drug group) for that drug; i.e., for naloxone, $N = 14$; methylnaloxonium chloride, $N = 15$; naltrexone, $N = 9$; naltrexone, $N = 9$; naltrexone methobromide, $N = 11$. Each dose consists of five separate observations. (From Koob et al., ref. 17, with permission.)

opiates has focused largely on the origin and projections of the medial forebrain bundle, a system implicated as a possible common neural substrate for the reinforcing properties of many drugs (18). For example, rats will self-administer morphine into the ventral tegmental area (VTA) (5), and other studies have shown that rats will directly self-administer morphine (24) and D-ala²-methionine enkephalin into the nucleus accumbens (n. acc.) (10). Indeed, Bozarth and Wise (4) have hypothesized that the mesolimbic dopamine (DA) system projecting within these regions is critical for the reinforcing properties of opiates. The next series of studies was designed to extend these observations by examining the effects of methylnaloxonium chloride (MN) on intravenous heroin self-administration after microinjection into the cerebral ventricles, the VTA, or n. acc.

The results showed that lateral ventricular injections of MN produced a dose-dependent increase in heroin self-administration similar to that observed for systemic injections of naloxone (Fig. 4). Effective doses ranged from 1.0 to 4.0 μg (for details see ref. 38). Similar results were obtained following injections of MN into the VTA with no effect of MN until reaching a dose of 1.0 μg. However, MN injected into the n. acc. was approximately eight-fold more potent at increasing self-administration of heroin. Significant increases were observed in doses as low as 0.125 to 0.25 μg with peak effects at 0.5 μg (Fig. 5) (for details see ref. 37).

Following completion of MN testing, rats injected in the n. acc. were switched from heroin to cocaine reward. After stable responding was established for cocaine

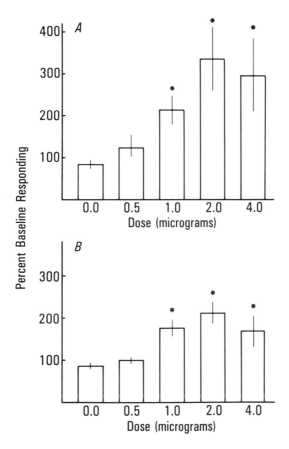

FIG. 4. The effects of intracerebroventricular methylnaloxonium chloride treatment on responding for heroin over the first hour (**A**) and over the total 3-hr self-administration session (**B**). Response rates were expressed as the percentage of baseline responding. *Asterisks* indicate that the treatment dose was significantly different from the saline treatment, *p* < 0.05, Newman-Keuls test. Six rats were tested across all drug treatments. The day prior to intracerebroventricular injections was used as the baseline day. (From Vaccarino et al., ref. 38, with permission.)

(0.75 mg/kg/injection), these rats received intra-n. acc. microinjections of 0.5 μg MN (optimal dose) 10 min prior to the self-administration session. MN had no effect on cocaine self-administration.

These overall results suggest that the n. acc. is an important and possibly critical substrate for the reinforcing actions of opiates. Effective doses of MN in the n. acc. were approximately eight times lower than those observed for lateral ventricular injections. Injections of MN into the VTA were no more effective than lateral ventricular injections and produced effects at doses similar to those used by others with quaternary nalorphine (6). One possibility is that the receptors critical for opiate reinforcement may be localized on the DA projections to the region of the n. acc. However, the persistence of opiate self-administration following destruction of these terminals with 6-hydroxydopamine (6-OHDA) (Pettit et al., 1984) suggests that the critical opiate receptors may be postsynaptic to the DA terminals.

The hypotheses that specific subtypes of opiate receptors may be involved in the reinforcing properties of opiates is a question of significant interest to pharmacologists (45) but a question difficult to address because of technical limitations

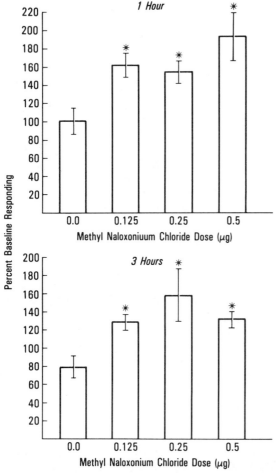

FIG. 5. Percent baseline (predrug day) responding for intravenous heroin during the first hour (*top graph*) and for the total 3 hr (*bottom graph*) of the heroin self-administration session following methyl-naloxonium chloride injections into the ventral tegmental area. *Asterisks* indicate a significant difference ($p < 0.05$) from both saline vehicle (0.0 dose) and 0.5 µg methylnaloxonium chloride. Duncan Multiple Range A Posteriori test. (From Vaccarino et al., ref. 37, with permission.)

as noted above. A variety of opiate drugs are self-administered by animals, including, in rats, morphine, codeine, etonitazene, meperidine, propoxyphene, as well as the mixed agonist-antagonist butorphanol, nalbuphine, nalorphine, and pentazocine (7). The opiate antagonists cyclazocine and naloxone were inactive, but ethylketazocine had clear reinforcing effects in rats (7) but not in monkeys (42). However, because of different pharmacokinetic characteristics of these drugs any correlation of potency for self-administration with binding affinity to opiate subtype would be meaningless. An alternative approach has been to examine the reinforcing efficacy of opiate agonists more or less specific to a given opiate receptor and from these data to generate hypotheses regarding a possible subtype of opiate receptor particularly involved in opiate reinforcement.

A number of opiate drugs when paired as unconditioned stimuli to a particular environment show the capability of imparting to that environment a positive reinforcing property (1,22,23,34,35). The measure of reinforcement in this paradigm is the return of the animal in a choice situation to the environment previously paired with the drug, i.e., a preference for that environment over an unpaired environment. Analogous to the classic taste preference procedures used by Wikler and associates in dependent rats (41), animals who are not physically dependent will show readily such a conditioned place preference with as few as one prior pairing with a drug such as heroin (22). In a recent study (21), the reinforcing efficacy of various opioid agonists acting preferentially on the κ and μ opioid receptors was assessed using the place preference conditioning paradigm. κ receptor agonists such as U50-488 and (−)bremazocine produced place aversions, whereas μ agonists such as morphine, fentanyl, and sufentanil produced place preferences (21).

Other experiments were directed at examining the reinforcing properties of β-endorphin (BEND) using a discrete trial, conditioned place preference test. BEND binds preferentially to μ and δ opiate receptor subtypes. The paradigm paired an intracerebroventricular injection of an opioid peptide with one distinctly different environment and saline with another distinct environment on alternate days for 6 days (training). Peptide injections were paired with the least preferred environment based on the preference of the rats in a pretreatment session; however, there were no overall differences in group preference before training. BEND (1.5, 2.5, 5.0, 10.0 μg/rat) was injected intracerebroventricularly (i.c.v. 2 μl volume) immediately before the rat was placed in the training box (for 30 min). Control rats were injected with either saline, morphine (10 μg i.c.v.), or heroin (0.5 mg/kg s.c.). After training, each rat was tested drug-free in a double-environment box where each end was identical to the training environments, with a smaller gray neutral area in the center. Time spent in each end of the test box was recorded over a 10-min period.

In a separate experiment, rats were similarly treated except that they received only one pairing of intracerebroventricular endorphin (2.5 μg) to the least preferred environment plus a subcutaneous injection of 0.04, 0.20, and 1.0 mg/kg of naloxone.

Heroin (0.5 mg/kg s.c.) produced strong preference for the heroin-paired environment. Rats also showed dose-dependent place preference for the environment paired with BEND (Fig. 6). Rats injected with the higher doses showed no preference for the paired environment but did show catalepsy and immobility with BEND (1). Naloxone effectively blocked this place preference at a dose as low as 0.04 mg/kg (Fig. 7). This dose had no effect on its own, but higher doses of naloxone alone produced a place aversion (M. Amalric et al., *unpublished results*, 1986).

These results demonstrate positive reinforcing properties for BEND. Given that BEND interacts mainly with μ and δ receptors, these results combined with the results with other selective opiate agonists (21) suggest that μ and δ receptors are the opiate receptor subtypes important for opiate reinforcement.

Further support for this hypothesis has been obtained using the self-admin-

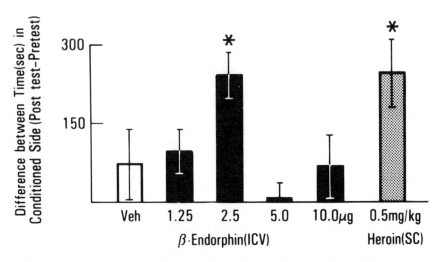

FIG. 6. The effects of intraventricular injections of β-endorphin on place preference in the rat. Data represent mean ± SEM of the difference in time between pretest and posttest on the conditioned side during a 10-min test after 6 days of conditioning (3 days β-endorphin on the paired side alternating with 3 days saline on the unpaired side). There was no systematic preference for the white or black side prior to training. Heroin was injected subcutaneously. *Significantly different from saline, Student's t-test.

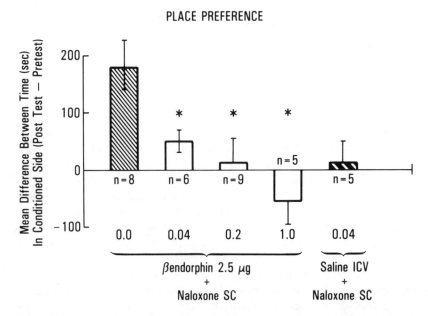

FIG. 7. The effects of naloxone injected systemically subcutaneously on place preference produced by intracerebroventricular injection of β-endorphin. Data represent mean ± SEM of the difference in time between pretest and posttest on the conditioned side during a 10-min test after 2 days of conditioning. *Significantly different from β-endorphin, Student's t-test.

istration procedure. As discussed above, many opiate agonists and mixed agonist-antagonists are self-administered by rats and monkeys. However, in rats, at least one study has found the putative κ agonist ethylketazocine to have reinforcing properties (7), even though it does not produce place preference or aversions.

To examine this question further, rats prepared with intravenous catheters and trained to self-administer heroin were subjected to a series of acute treatments with μ and κ agonists during self-administration. Following establishment of a dose-dependent pause in opiate self-administration, verification of the ability of a given compound to substitute for heroin was obtained by replacing the heroin with the drug in question.

Six rats were allowed to self-administer heroin for 3 hr/day on a fixed ratio (FR) 5 Schedule of Reinforcement. During response pause testing the rats were allowed 1 hr access to heroin; they were then removed and injected with 0.01, 0.02, or 0.04 mg/kg of fentanyl (μ agonist) or 0.25, 0.50, or 1.0 mg/kg of U50-488 (κ agonist). Following each series the respective agonists were substituted as the drug to be self-administered at a dose deemed equivalent to that used for heroin.

As can be seen in Table 2, fentanyl produced a dose-dependent pause in self-administration when injected subcutaneously during a heroin self-administration test. Fentanyl also readily substituted for heroin on a subsequent test day at a dose of 0.006 mg/kg/injection. U50-488 failed to produce any systematic response pauses in doses as high as 1.0 mg/kg and failed to substitute for heroin at a dose of 0.15 mg/kg/injection on a subsequent trial. These results suggest that the reinforcing properties of heroin are related to an activation of the μ opiate receptor subtype.

Cocaine

Catecholamines have been strongly implicated in the reinforcing properties of psychomotor stimulants (26). More specifically, the reinforcing properties of psychomotor stimulants have been linked to the activation of central DA neurons and their postsynaptic receptors. When the synthesis of catecholamines is inhibited by administering α-methyl-para-tyrosine, an attenuation of the reinforcing effects of psychomotor stimulants occurs (25a; 16). Furthermore, low doses of DA antagonists will increase the response rates for intravenous injections of *d*-amphetamine and cocaine (8,9,44). It was hypothesized that a partial blockade of DA receptors produced a partial blockade of the reinforcing effects of these indirect sympathomimetics. Thus, animals are thought to compensate for decreases in the magnitude of the reinforcer by increasing their self-administration behavior (see above and Fig. 2).

The role of dopamine in the reinforcing properties of cocaine was extended by the observation that 6-OHDA lesions of the n. acc. produce extinction-like responding and a significant and long-lasting reduction in self-administration of cocaine over days (19,30,32). Similar decreases in cocaine self-administration were observed in rats with lesions of the VTA (31). While these decreases in self-administration suggest a decrease in the reinforcing efficacy of cocaine, not all rats showed a clear extinction-like pattern of responding, leaving open the possibility of alternative nonmotivational interpretations. Thus, to confirm that the lesion deficit was motivational and to examine the anatomical specificity of this effect, separate groups of rats trained to a stable baseline of cocaine self-administration were subjected to 6-OHDA lesions of the n. acc. or corpus striatum. Postlesion, the rats were tested for 3 days on the training dose of cocaine 0.75 mg/kg injection and then were subjected to a dose-effect determination where the dose of cocaine was halved, returned to normal (0.75 mg/kg/injection), and then doubled on 3 successive days. Following this, a progressive ratio schedule probe was administered over a 6-hr period. The rats were allowed access to heroin, but on every injection the response requirement was augmented by one step (Table 3).

The results showed a decrease in responding for cocaine during the first 3 days postlesion in the rats with 6-OHDA lesions to the n. acc., as has been previously reported (Fig. 8, top). A similar decrease in responding was observed at all doses in the dose-effect function, although the effect was much more dramatic at the highest dose, resulting in a generally flat dose-effect function in the rats with 6-OHDA lesions (Fig. 8, middle). In contrast, there was no effect on response rate in the rats with 6-OHDA lesions of the corpus striatum.

TABLE 2. *Effects of fentanyl and U50-488 on heroin self-administration in the rat*

	Response pause (min)[a]		Self-administration (number infusions)[a]
Fentanyl		Fentanyl (0.006 mg/kg/injection)	
0	10.0 ± 1.3^{b}	Total 3 hours	15.2 ± 2.4
0.01 mg/kg	33.7 ± 5.9	1st hour	6.7 ± 0.7
0.02 mg/kg	51.5 ± 7.8	2nd hour	4.5 ± 1.0
0.04 mg/kg	74.0 ± 7.6	3rd hour	4.0 ± 0.9
U50-488		U50-488 (0.15 mg/kg/injection)	
0	10.0 ± 1.3^{b}	Total 3 hours	5.5 ± 1.7
0.25 mg/kg	17.2 ± 2.9	1st hour	4.5 ± 1.4
0.50 mg/kg	36.8 ± 15.0	2nd hour	0.5 ± 0.5
1.00 mg/kg	$13.0 \pm 2.,5$	3rd hour	0.5 ± 0.3
Heroin		Heroin (0.06 mg/kg/injection)	
0	10.0 ± 1.3^{b}	Total 3 hours	16 ± 1.9
0.1 mg/kg	21.3 ± 6.8	1st hour	7.2 ± 0.9
0.2 mg/kg	43.0 ± 11.9	2nd hour	5.0 ± 0.7
0.4 mg/kg	65.2 ± 10.9	3rd hour	3.8 ± 0.7
		Saline	
		Total 3 hours	6.0 ± 1.9
		1st hour	4.5 ± 2.1
		2nd hour	0.0 ± 0.0
		3rd hour	0.3 ± 0.2

[a] Values represent mean ± SEM for 6 rats.
[b] Represents the same observations for a single systemic saline injection 1 hr into a 3-hr heroin self-administration session.

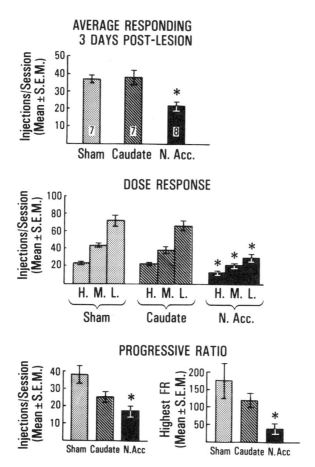

FIG. 8. Effects of 6-hydroxydopamine (6-OHDA) lesions to the nucleus accumbens and corpus striatum on responding for rats self-administering cocaine. *Top panel* shows continuous reinforcement data averaged over the first 3 days postlesion (means ± SEM). Sham, vehicle (0.1 mg/ml ascorbic acid in saline) injected controls. Caudate, rats receiving 8 μg in 2 μl of 6-OHDA injected into the corpus striatum. N. acc., rats receiving 8 μg in 2 μl of 6-OHDA injected into the nucleus accumbens. *Middle panel* shows the dose-effect functions for each group. H, 2 times the normal 0.75 mg/kg/injection dose; M refers to middle dose range, 0.75 mg/kg/injection; L refers to one-half of the 0.75 mg/kg/injection dose. *Bottom panel* shows the mean rewards and mean highest ratio obtained by each group on the progressive ratio probe. *Significantly different from sham group. $p < 0.05$ Newman–Keuls test.

The results from the progressive ratio probe supported the hypothesis that these decreases in response rate reflected a decrease in the reinforcing properties of cocaine. 6-OHDA lesions of the n. acc. dramatically decreased the FR value for which the rats would continue to work (Fig. 8, bottom). A smaller, not statistically reliable decrease was observed in the rats with corpus striatum lesions. These results suggest that depletion of DA in the n. acc. can significantly decrease the reinforcing value of cocaine.

TABLE 3. *Progressive ratio schedule*

Day 1	6 hr continuous reinforcement	
Day 2	6 hr progressive increase in fixed ratio	
Reinforcer number in sequence	Increment in FR per reinforcer	Requirement per reinforcer/, i.e., FR value
1–8	+1	1–8
9–16	+2	10–24
17–24	+4	28–56
25–32	+8	64–120
32+, after each reinforcer FR incremented 8 responses		

These results demonstrated that postsynaptic blockade of DA receptors or destruction of presynaptic DA terminals in the region of the n. acc. significantly decreased the reinforcing value of psychomotor stimulants. Thus, the mesolimbic DA system appears to be critical for psychomotor stimulant reinforcement (19,30,32).

In summary, drugs can function as consequence events (reinforcers) in establishing and controlling operant behavior. The self-administration procedure in animals, including rodents, has proven to be a reliable indicator of the abuse liability of drugs. Drug self-administration also has advantages as a procedure for measuring the reinforcing value of drugs, because many of the classical operant techniques can be applied to measure the motivational value of the drug as well as the relative reinforcement value of the drug. Self-administration is also useful in the pharmacology of drug action because of reproducible and orderly dose-effect functions and antagonism interactions. Finally, animal drug self-administration is particularly useful for delineation of the neurobiological site and mechanism of action for the reinforcing properties of drugs. As an example, evidence is presented summarizing work aimed at determining the neurochemical substrates for the reinforcing properties of opiates and psychomotor stimulants in rats who are not physically dependent. Systemic injections of naloxone and intracerebral injections of its less lipophilic quaternary analog methylnaloxonium into the region of the n. acc. shift dose-effect functions for heroin self-administration to the right. Lesions of the presynaptic DA input to the n. acc. significantly attenuate cocaine and amphetamine self-administration measured either with response rate or a progressive ratio schedule. Results suggest that the n. acc. and its connections may play an important role in the neurobiology of drug reinforcement.

REFERENCES

1. Amalric, M., Martinez, Jr., J. L., Ling, N., Bloom, F. E., and Koob, G. F. (1986): Rewarding properties of β-endorphins as measured by conditioned place preference. *Psychopharmacology* (*in press*).

2. Bedford, J. A., Bailey, L. P., and Wilson, M. C. (1978): Cocaine reinforced progressive ratio performance in the rhesus monkey. *Pharmacol. Biochem. Behav.,* 9:631–638.
3. Bianchi, G., Fiocchi, R., Tavani, A., and Manara, L. (1982): Quaternary narcotic antagonists' relative ability to prevent antinociception and gastrointestinal transit inhibition in morphine treated rats as an index of peripheral selectivity. *Life Sci.,* 30:1875–1883.
4. Bozarth, M. A., and Wise, R. A. (1981): Heroin reward is dependent on a dopaminergic substrate. *Life Sci.,* 29:1881–1886.
5. Bozarth, M. A., and Wise, R. A. (1981): Intracranial self-administration of morphine into the ventral tegmental area in rats. *Life Sci.,* 28:551–555.
6. Britt, M. D., and Wise, R. A. (1983): Ventral tegmental site of opiate reward: Antagonism by a hydrophilic opiate receptor blocker. *Brain Res.,* 258:105–108.
7. Collins, R. J., Weeks, J. R., Cooper, M. M., Good, P. I., and Russell, R. R. (1984): Prediction of abuse liability of drugs using IV self-administration by rats. *Psychopharmacology (Berlin),* 82: 6–13.
8. Davis, W. M., and Smith, S. G. (1975): Effect of haloperidol on (+)-amphetamine self-administration. *J. Pharmacy Pharmacol.,* 27:540–542.
9. Ettenberg, A., Pettit, H. O., Bloom, F. E., and Koob, G. F. (1982): Heroin and cocaine self-administration in rats: Mediation by separate neural systems. *Psychopharmacology (Berlin),* 78: 204–209.
10. Goeders, N. E., Lane, T. D., and Smith, J. E. (1984): Self-administration of methionine enkephalin into the nucleus accumbens. *Pharmacol. Biochem. Behav.,* 20:451–455.
11. Goldberg, S. R., Woods, J. H., and Schuster, C. R. (1971): Nalorphine-induced changes in morphine self-administration rhesus monkeys. *J. Pharmacol. Exp. Ther.,* 176:464–471.
12. Griffiths, R. R., Bigelow, G. E., and Henningfield, J. E. (1980): Similarities in animal and human drug-taking behavior. In: *Advances in Substance Abuse, Vol. 1,* edited by N. K. Mello, pp. 1–90. JAI, Greenwich, Connecticut.
13. Griffiths, R. R., Brady, J. V., and Snell, J. D. (1978): Progressive-ratio performance maintained by drug infusions: Comparison of cocaine, diethylpropion, chlorphentermine, and fenfluramine. *Psychopharmacology (Berlin),* 56:5–13.
14. Griffiths, R. R., Findley, J. A., Brady, J. V., Guther, K., and Robinson, W. (1975): Comparison of progressive ratio performance maintained by cocaine, methylphenidate and secobarbital. *Psychopharmacologia,* 43:81–83.
15. Jaffe, J. H. (1980): Drug addiction and drug abuse. In: *Goodman and Gilman's the Pharmacological Basis of Therapeutics,* edited by L. S. Goodman, A. Gilman, A. E. Mayer, and K. L. Melmon, pp. 545–546. MacMillan Publishing Company, New York.
16. Jonsson, L. E., Anggard, E., and Gunne, L. M. (1971): Blockade of intravenous amphetamine euphoria in man. *Clin. Pharmacol. Ther.,* 12:889–896.
17. Koob, G. F., Pettit, H. O., Ettenberg, A., and Bloom, F. E. (1984): Effects of opiate antagonists and their quaternary derivatives on heroin self-administration in the rat. *J. Pharmacol. Exp. Ther.,* 229:481–486.
18. Kornetsky, C., Esposito, R. U., McLean, S., and Jacobson, J. O. (1979): Intracranial self-stimulation thresholds: A model for the hedonic effects of drugs of abuse. *Arch. Gen. Psychiatry,* 36:289–292.
19. Lyness, W. H., Friedle, N. M., and Moore, K. E. (1979): Destruction of dopaminergic nerve terminals in nucleus accumbens: Effect of *d*-amphetamine self-administration. *Pharmacol. Biochem. Behav.,* 11:663–666.
20. Meyer, R. E., and Mirin, S. M. (1979): *The Heroin Stimulus.* Plenum Medical Book Company, New York.
21. Mucha, R. F., and Herz, A. (1985): Motivational properties of kappa and mu opioid receptor agonists studied with place and taste preference conditioning. *Psychopharmacology (Berlin),* 86: 274–280.
22. Mucha, R. F., and Iversen, S. D. (1984): Reinforcing properties of morphine and naloxone revealed by conditioned place preferences: A procedural examination. *Psychopharmacology (Berlin),* 82:241–247.
23. Mucha, R. F., van der Kooy, D., O'Shaughnessy, M., and Bucenieks, P. (1982): Drug reinforcement studied by use of place conditioning in rats. *Brain Res.,* 243:91–105.
24a. Pettit, H. O., Ettenberg, A., Bloom, F. E., and Loob, G. F. (1984): Destruction of the nucleus

accumbens selectively attenuates cocaine but not heroin self-administration in rats. *Psychopharmacology (Berlin)*, 54:167–173.
25. Pickens, R., and Harris, W. C. (1968): Self-administration of d-amphetamine by rats. *Psychopharmacologia,* 12:158–163.
25a.Pickens, R., Mersch, R. A., and Dougherty, J. A. (1968): Chemical interactions in methamphetamine reinforcement. *Psychol. Rep.,* 23:1267–1270.
26. Pickens, R., Meisch, R. A., and Thompson, J. (1978): Drug self-administration An analysis of the reinforcing effects of drugs. In: *Handbook of Psychopharmacology, Vol. 12,* edited by L. L. Iversen, S. D. Iversen, and S. H. Snyder, pp. 1–37. Plenum Press, New York.
27. Pickens, R., and Thompson, T. (1968): Cocaine reinforced behavior in rats: Effects of reinforcement magnitude and fixed ratio size. *J. Pharmacol. Exp. Ther.,* 161:122–129.
28. Risner, M. E., and Goldberg, S. R. (1983): A comparison of nicotine and cocaine self-administration in the dog: Fixed ratio and progressive ratio schedules of intravenous drug infusion. *J. Pharmacol. Exp. Ther.,* 224:319–326.
29. Risner, M. E., and Silcox, D. L. (1981): Psychostimulant self-administration by beagle dogs in a progressive-ratio paradigm. *Psychopharmacology (Berlin),* 75:25–30.
30. Roberts, D. C. S., Corcoran, M. E., and Fibiger, H. C. (1977): On the role of ascending catecholaminergic systems in intravenous self-administration of cocaine. *Pharmacol. Biochem. Behav.,* 6:615–620.
31. Roberts, D. C. S., and Koob, G. F. (1982): Disruption of cocaine self-administration following 6-hydroxydopamine lesions of the central tegmental area in rats. *Pharmacol. Biochem. Behav.,* 17:901–904.
32. Roberts, D. C. S., Koob, G. F., Klonoff, P., and Fibiger, H. C. (1980): Extinction and recovery of cocaine self-administration following 6-hydroxydopamine lesions of the nucleus accumbens. *Pharmacol. Biochem. Behav.,* 12:781–787.
33. Schuster, C. R., and Thompson, T. (1969): Self-administration of and behavioral dependence on drug. *Annu. Rev. Pharmacol. Toxicol.,* 9:483–502.
34. Spyraki, C., Fibiger, H. C., and Phillips, A. G. (1983): Attenuation of heroin reward in rats by destruction of the mesolimbic dopamine system. *Psychopharmacology (Berlin),* 79:278–283.
35. Stolerman, I. P., Pilcher, C. W., and D'Mello, G. D. (1978): Stereospecific aversion property of narcotic antagonists in morphine-free rats. *Life Sci.,* 22:1755–1762.
36. Tavani, A., Bianchi, G., and Manara, L. (1979): Morphine no longer blocks gastrointestinal transit but retains antinociceptive action in diallyl-normorphine-pretreated rats. *Eur. J. Pharmacol.,* 59:151–154.
37. Vaccarino, F. J., Bloom, F. E., and Koob, G. F. (1985): Blockade of nucleus accumbens opiate receptors attenuates intravenous heroin reward in the rat. *Psychopharmacology (Berlin),* 86:37–42.
38. Vaccarino, F. J., Pettit, H. O., Bloom, F. E., and Koob, G. F. (1985): Effects of intracerebroventricular administration of methylnaloxone chloride on heroin self-administration in the rat. *Pharmacol. Biochem. Behav.,* 23:495–498.
39. Weeks, J. R. (1962): Experimental morphine addiction: Method for automatic intravenous injections in unrestrained rats. *Science,* 138:143–144.
40. Weeks, J. R., and Collins, R. J. (1976): Changes in morphine self-administration in rats induced by prostaglandin E and naloxone. *Prostaglandins,* 12:11–19.
41. Wikler, A. (1965): Narcotics. In: *Conditioning Factors in Opiate Addictions and Relapse,* edited by D. M. Wilner and G. G. Kassebaum, pp. 85–100. McGraw-Hill Book Company, New York.
42. Woods, J. H., Smith, C. B., Medzihradsky, F., and Swain, H. H. (1979): Preclinical testing of new analgesic drugs. In: *Mechanisms of Pain and Analgesic Compounds,* edited by R. E. Beers and E. G. Bassett, pp. 429–445. Raven Press, New York.
43. Yanagita, T. (1973): An experimental framework for evaluations of dependence liability of various types of drugs in monkeys. *Bull. Narc.,* 25:57–64.
44. Yokel, R. A., and Wise, R. A. (1976): Attenuation of intravenous amphetamine reinforcement by central dopamine blockade in rats. *Psychopharmacology (Berlin),* 48:311–318.
45. Zukin, R. S., and Zukin, S. R. (1984): The case for multiple opiate receptors. *TINS,* 7:160–164.

Brain Reward Systems and Abuse, edited by
J. Engel and L. Oreland.
Raven Press, New York © 1987.

Cerebral Metabolic Changes Associated with Activation of Reward Systems

Linda J. Porrino[1]

Laboratory of Cerebral Metabolism, National Institute of Mental Health, Public Health
Service, Department of Health and Human Services, Bethesda, Maryland 20892

It is commonly believed that drugs of abuse achieve their reinforcing properties by interacting with reward systems in the brain. The phenomenon of intracranial self-stimulation (ICSS) has been long considered a productive means of studying these systems. ICSS was first demonstrated by Olds and Milner in 1954 (5) when they observed that rats would work in order to receive brief trains of electrical stimulation directly to certain brain sites. ICSS is commonly viewed as an artificial activation of the brain's normal positive reinforcement mechanisms and as such can be used as a model of goal-directed or reinforced behavior. This view is supported by the fact that the characteristics of responding for brain stimulation are identical to the ways in which animals respond for natural rewards such as food and water (5,6,22). A central problem in the study of ICSS has been the identification of the neural circuits activated during this behavior. Although many different methods have been applied to this problem, this report will focus on the application of the quantitative 2-deoxyglucose autoradiographic method to the characterization of the anatomical substrates of rewarded behavior.

The development by Sokoloff and colleagues of the 2-[^{14}C]deoxyglucose (2-DG) method affords a novel opportunity to map functional neural pathways simultaneously in all anatomical components of the CNS of conscious animals (19). It is based on the close relationship between the level of energy metabolism (in the brain, glucose is virtually the exclusive substrate for energy metabolism) and the level of functional activity. It is possible to map local regions of altered functional activity in the brain during pharmacological or behavioral manipulations by measurement of changes in rates of local cerebral glucose utilization (LCGU) in these structures (19). A radioactive labeled analog of glucose, 2-DG, is used, which, like glucose, is transported into cerebral tissue and phosphorylated by hexokinase but, unlike glucose, is trapped within cells. Thus, quantitative autoradiography can be used, permitting not only the measurement of actual

---

[1] *Present address:* National Institutes on Drug Abuse, Addiction Research Center, Baltimore, Maryland 21224

rates of glucose utilization in individual brain regions but also a pictorial representation of the relative rates of glucose utilization throughout the entire brain. For detailed discussion of the theoretical bases of the method and reviews of some of its applications see Sokoloff (18) and Sokoloff et al. (19).

There have been two main experimental strategies in the application of the 2-DG method to the identification of brain reinforcement circuits. The first approach involves the use of ICSS as a model of reinforced behavior. In these studies, electrodes are placed in a variety of different brain sites that support ICSS, and the alterations in LCGU that result from stimulation at each site are measured. By comparing the similarities and the differences in the patterns of changes in local cerebral energy metabolism that are associated with ICSS at different anatomical sites, the question of common anatomical substrates of ICSS can be addressed. Early work using this basic approach, however, was not very fruitful (4,23). A study comparing animals self-stimulating to the medial forebrain bundle, prefrontal cortex, and the locus ceruleus failed to detect any consistent changes in deoxyglucose uptake in any brain region (23). Because a nonquantitative modification of the 2-DG method was used in this work, only relative rates of glucose utilization could be estimated, and the analysis was thereby limited to side-to-side comparisons within the same animal. In order to be able to accurately detect differences in rates of LCGU across animals in different experimental conditions or physiologic states, especially those changes that are not limited to one side of the brain or the other, the fully quantitative version of the 2-DG method should be used. Using relative rates, only the very largest differences can be seen and only comparisons between sides of the brain can be made with any confidence. In contrast, by using the fully quantitative version of the method, as has been done in the studies described in the following sections, even subtle changes that occur bilaterally can be measured with precision.

The second approach involves the administration of drugs that are known to act as reinforcers or can alter the reinforcement value of brain stimulation. The examination and comparison of the changes in local brain energy metabolism that are associated with the drug-treated and untreated conditions can provide information about the neural substrates of drug action.

MAPPING STUDIES

Intracranial Self-Stimulation to the Ventral Tegmental Area

In a series of experiments using the first approach, we have defined the pattern of changes in local cerebral glucose utilization that accompanies ICSS to the ventral tegmental area (VTA). In this first study (3), rates of glucose utilization of freely moving rats working for rewarding brain stimulation to the VTA were compared to rates in passive control rats that had electrodes aimed at the VTA but were not stimulated. Results revealed a selective pattern of metabolic activation in the terminal fields of the VTA, including such areas as the medial prefrontal cortex, portions of the amygdala, nucleus accumbens, mediodorsal nucleus of the thalamus, and the locus ceruleus (Fig. 1). Significant increases in metabolic activity were seen as well in various sensory and motor structures involved in the performance of lever-pressing task itself. Self-stimulation to the VTA involves the activation of a selective, discretely organized neural system with representations at all levels of the neuraxis.

The essence of reinforced behavior is the contingent association between the response and its consequences—in the case of ICSS, the lever press and the brain stimulation. A stimulus, such as brain stimulation, cannot be considered reinforcing unless it can be shown that a contingent relationship between behavior and administration of the stimulus can be demonstrated (14). In fact, rats learn to escape response-independent presentation of electrical brain stimulation for which they had previously worked (21). In order to isolate the neural circuits associated with the contingent presentation of electrical stimulation to the VTA that are, therefore, directly related to reinforcement, we compared rates of glucose utilization in three groups of rats: (a) animals self-stimulating to the VTA; (b) animals receiving experimenter-administered electrical stimulation (EAS) to the VTA at rates and parameters for which they had previously self-stimulated; and (c) animals receiving no stimulation (10). Both the ICSS and the EAS groups showed a similar pattern of metabolic activation, as assessed by changes in LCGU, at the stimulation site and in the direct rostral and caudal projection fibers in the medial forebrain bundle and pontine gray, respectively (Table 1). The pattern of alterations in local metabolic rates in ICSS and EAS animals were divergent, however, in the terminal fields of the VTA. There were extensive changes in glucose utilization in the ICSS animals that were not present in the EAS group. These included bilateral increases in the nucleus accumbens, lateral septum, hippocampus, mediodorsal thalamus, and the locus ceruleus (Table 1). In addition, side-to-side differences were seen in the amygdala and medial prefrontal cortex in the ICSS group but not in the EAS group (Table 1). The widespread distribution of changes in metabolic activity found in the self-stimulating animals should be considered specific to the reinforced behavior of these animals and not merely the result of the electrical stimulation of the VTA.

Intracranial Self-Stimulation to the Substantia Nigra

A similar series of experiments was carried out in rats with electrodes in the substantia nigra pars compacta (SN), an area anatomically continuous with the VTA in the ventral midbrain (8). Three groups of animals were also used: (a) ICSS, (b) EAS, and (c) no stimulation. Both the ICSS and EAS groups showed a similar pattern of metabolic activation, as assessed by changes in LCGU, at the stimulation site and in the direct rostral and caudal projections (Table 2).

A

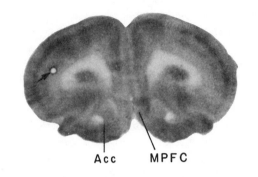

A10500

B

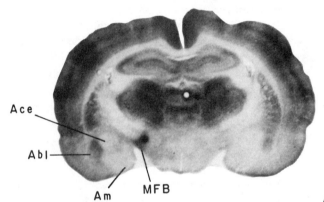

A4620

C

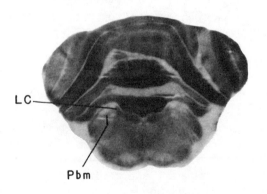

P1500

TABLE 1. *Effects of ventral tegmental area stimulation on local cerebral glucose utilization (mean μmol/100 g/min ± SEM)*

Structure	No Stimulation (N = 5)		Experimenter-Administered Stimulation (N = 5)		Self-Stimulation (N = 5)	
	Ipsi.	Contra.	Ipsi.	Contra.	Ipsi.	Contra.
Ventral tegmental area	59 ± 4	59 ± 4	182 ± 10[a,b]	88 ± 3	189 ± 11[a,b]	95 ± 7
Medial forebrain bundle	60 ± 2	59 ± 2	103 ± 6[a,b]	72 ± 4	116 ± 7[a,b]	77 ± 2
Pontine gray	60 ± 2	59 ± 3	105 ± 5[a,b]	86 ± 5	110 ± 11[a,b]	86 ± 7
Nucleus accumbens	82 ± 4	83 ± 4	88 ± 3	87 ± 3	98 ± 2[a]	97 ± 3
Caudate (ventrolateral)	99 ± 5	99 ± 5	101 ± 6	101 ± 5	113 ± 7	109 ± 6
Lateral septum	58 ± 3	59 ± 2	76 ± 4[b]	64 ± 3	74 ± 3[a]	71 ± 3
Amygdala (central)	42 ± 1	43 ± 1	46 ± 3	43 ± 1	51 ± 2[b]	46 ± 2
Medial prefrontal cortex	81 ± 3	82 ± 2	74 ± 3	69 ± 3	98 ± 3[b]	85 ± 3
Anterior cingulate cortex	98 ± 5	97 ± 5	106 ± 3	103 ± 3	99 ± 3	103 ± 4
Mediodorsal thalamus	100 ± 5	100 ± 6	119 ± 6[b]	110 ± 5	129 ± 6[a]	127 ± 6
Hippocampus (CA3)	70 ± 4	72 ± 4	87 ± 3[b]	80 ± 3	93 ± 4[a]	89 ± 3
Locus ceruleus	66 ± 4	65 ± 4	87 ± 5[a]	82 ± 4	93 ± 4[a,b]	76 ± 4

[a] Combined ipsilateral and contralateral values differ from the combined ipsilateral and contralateral values in the no stimulation control group ($p < 0.05$).
[b] Difference between ipsilateral and contralateral values differs from the corresponding difference in the no stimulation control group ($p < 0.05$).
Ipsi., ipsilateral; Contra., contralateral.

There was an intense increase in LCGU at the stimulation site in the SN, which continued rostrally within the dorsolateral aspect of the medial forebrain bundle, extending to the lateral preoptic area. Caudal to the stimulation site there were LCGU increases in the projection fibers extending through the pontine gray.

The pattern of LCGU changes within cortical and striatal terminal fields and major striatal outflow pathways, however, was distinctly different in the ICSS and EAS groups (Table 2). Bilateral increases in LCGU relative to the unstimulated group were found, for example, in the caudate (all aspects), anterior cin-

FIG. 1. Autoradiographs of coronal brain sections from three self-stimulating rats at various rostral-caudal levels. Glucose utilization is a function of optical density. *Arrows* point to artifacts due to tissue processing. A: Level of the rostral forebrain. There is a small area of increased optical density in the right medial prefrontal cortex, ipsilateral to the site of stimulation, that extends across cortical layers but extends ventrally and dorsally most prominently in the innermost layers of the cortex. B: Level of the diencephalon. The circumscribed area of high optical density in the left lateral medial forebrain bundle is the bundle of activated fibers extending from the ventral tegmental area electrode site. Note asymmetries in the optical densities of the nuclei of the amygdala. Increases are most evident in the basolateral nucleus of the amygdala on the left, ipsilateral to the stimulated electrode. C: Level of the pons. On the left, ipsilateral to the electrode site, a higher optical density is apparent in the locus ceruleus. Note punctate distribution of densities in the cerebellar hemispheres. This pattern is consistent with the motor activity of the animal during the experiment. Abl, basolateral amygdaloid nucleus; Acc, nucleus accumbens; Ace, central amygdaloid nucleus; Am, medial amygdaloid nucleus; LC, locus ceruleus; MFB, medial forebrain bundle; MPFC, medial prefrontal cortex; Pbm, medial parabrachial nucleus. (From Esposito et al., ref. 3, with permission.)

TABLE 2. *Effects of substantia nigra stimulation on local cerebral glucose utilization*
(mean μmol/100 g/min ± SEM)

Structure	No Stimulation (N = 5)		Experimenter-Administered Stimulation (N = 5)		Self-Stimulation (N = 5)	
	Ipsi.	Contra.	Ipsi.	Contra.	Ipsi.	Contra.
Substantia nigra pars compacta	66 ± 3	69 ± 4	>250[a,b]	82 ± 3	<250[a,b]	97 ± 4
Caudate (dorsomedial)	106 ± 4	106 ± 4	112 ± 7	109 ± 7	139 ± 6[a,b]	130 ± 6
Caudate (ventrolateral)	92 ± 2	93 ± 4	113 ± 9[b]	106 ± 10	139 ± 5[a,b]	120 ± 3
Globus pallidus	55 ± 3	55 ± 3	76 ± 4[b]	54 ± 5	93 ± 9[a]	77 ± 4
Anterior cingulate cortex	109 ± 5	108 ± 7	106 ± 8	105 ± 7	128 ± 2[a]	123 ± 3
Nucleus accumbens	79 ± 4	79 ± 3	82 ± 5	82 ± 4	106 ± 5[a]	103 ± 4
Medial prefrontal cortex	71 ± 4	73 ± 3	69 ± 5	67 ± 5	87 ± 2[a]	85 ± 1
Lateral septum	64 ± 5	65 ± 4	63 ± 5	60 ± 4	79 ± 3[a]	77 ± 3
Mediodorsal thalamus	103 ± 5	107 ± 6	123 ± 7	106 ± 3	141 ± 4[a]	137 ± 5

[a] Combined ipsilateral and contralateral values differ from the combined ipsilateral and contra-lateral values in the no stimulation control group ($p < 0.05$).
[b] Difference between ipsilateral and contralateral values differs from the corresponding difference in the no stimulation control group ($p < 0.05$).
Ipsi., ipsilateral; Contra., contralateral.

gulate cortex, and globus pallidus in the ICSS group. These areas were not activated or only unilaterally activated in EAS animals. Furthermore, changes were evident in areas that receive few direct anatomical projections from the SN, in particular, the medial prefrontal cortex and the nucleus accumbens in the ICSS group but not the EAS group when compared to unstimulated controls. As in animals receiving VTA stimulation contingent, response-dependent electrical stimulation resulted in far more extensive effects on metabolic activity than did noncontingent, response-independent EAS. Many of the same areas in which differences are seen in these studies using the 2-DG method with brain stimulation have been shown to be involved in reinforcement processes in studies of neurotransmitter turnover rates in brains of rats self-administering morphine and in yoked morphine-infused controls (15–17). This isomorphism of findings suggests that the behavioral context of stimulus presentation is a significant factor in determining the neurochemical effects of a variety of stimuli in the brain.

Comparison of Ventral Tegmental Area and Substantia Nigra Self-Stimulation

The SN and the VTA, although anatomically continuous within the ventral midbrain, have different afferent and efferent projections (cf. ref. 1). Behaviorally, ICSS to these areas is characterized by differences in response rate, threshold, and response topography (2,7,9). A direct comparison (8) of the distribution of LCGU changes accompanying ICSS to the SN and to the VTA revealed that in areas such as the hippocampus, olfactory tubercle, central amygdala, and bed nucleus of the stria terminalis, metabolic rates in animals self-stimulating to the

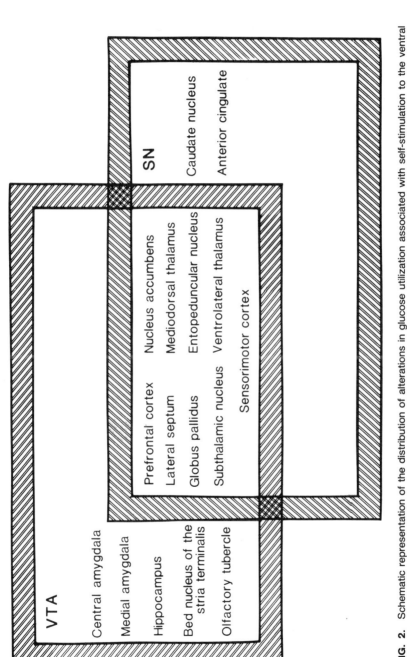

FIG. 2. Schematic representation of the distribution of alterations in glucose utilization associated with self-stimulation to the ventral tegmental area (VTA) and to the substantia nigra pars compacta (SN). Structures listed in *central rectangle* are those in which significant changes were seen in both self-stimulation groups.

VTA were significantly higher than in animals self-stimulating to the SN (Fig. 2). In contrast, rates of glucose utilization in the anterior cingulate and in the caudate were significantly higher in animals self-stimulating to the SN than those self-stimulating to the VTA (Fig. 2). The pattern of functional activity associated with ICSS to the VTA is, therefore, different from the pattern associated with ICSS to the SN. These data lend support to the concept of multiple neuronal systems underlying reinforcement.

When compared to unstimulated controls, the rates of metabolic activity in the thalamus, sensorimotor cortex, subthalamic nucleus, and cerebellar cortex of animals self-stimulating to the VTA as well as SN were significantly increased. In addition, rates of LCGU in these structures were higher in VTA animals than in SN animals. Such differences are noteworthy, because these are areas known to be involved in the production of motor responses. The self-stimulating animals are all lever-pressing but at different rates. Significant positive correlations were found between rates of lever-pressing and levels of glucose utilization in these structures. The relationship between rate of motor responding and rate of energy metabolism suggests that these areas are involved in the production of the lever-pressing itself and are not directly involved with reinforcement. There were, however, a core set of structures in which metabolic rates were similarly increased in both groups in an equivalent manner. These areas include the prefrontal cortex, nucleus accumbens, lateral septum, and the mediodorsal nucleus of the thalamus. This convergence of metabolic activation indicates that these are the regions central to the production and maintenance of positively reinforced behavior.

PHARMACOLOGICAL STUDIES

The 2-DG method has proved highly useful in determining the sites of action, both direct and indirect, of various pharmacological agents. For example, the method has been used to study the effects on rat cerebral energy metabolism of a frequently abused class of drugs, the psychostimulants, in doses comparable to those which are self-administered intravenously. Amphetamine (12) and methylphenidate at such doses (11) produce highly selective changes in glucose utilization confined to the nucleus accumbens. In contrast, the most prominent alteration in metabolic activity that accompanied acute cocaine administration occurred in the medial prefrontal cortex (L. J. Porrino, *unpublished observations*, 1985). Although all three psychostimulants affect the metabolic activity of regions innervated by neurons arising in the VTA, the cortical terminal fields were preferentially affected by cocaine, whereas limbic terminal fields were primarily affected by amphetamine and methylphenidate. On the basis of the differences in the distribution of alterations in energy metabolism, it can be concluded that these drugs may produce their behavioral effects through different anatomical paths.

It is well known that amphetamine pretreatment induces an increase in the rate of responding for ICSS (20). We have used the 2-DG method to look at the ways in which amphetamine affects rewarding brain stimulation. Four groups of animals were compared: (a) high-current ICSS, (b) low-current ICSS plus 0.5 mg/kg amphetamine, (c) 0.5 mg/kg amphetamine alone, and (d) no treatment. Animals in the high-current and in the low-current plus amphetamine groups had responded at the same rates. In this way, we could look at equivalent behavior produced in two different ways, either by pharmacological manipulation or by changes in the magnitude of the electrical stimulation. Rates of glucose utilization were lower at the stimulation site and pathway in the low-current group plus amphetamine than in the high-current group. Rates of metabolic activity were increased to an equivalent degree, however, in selected portions of the terminal fields of the VTA including the nucleus accumbens, lateral septum, and locus ceruleus. In the olfactory tubercle and caudate, glucose utilization was greater in the low-current plus amphetamine group than in the high-current group. Although these data are preliminary, they indicate, first, that metabolic changes in the stimulation pathways are related to the current intensity and, second, that equivalent response rates whether arising from high current levels or pharmacological manipulation yield strikingly similar patterns of glucose utilization changes in the terminal fields of the VTA. Amphetamine and brain stimulation, then, are activating the same neural reinforcement pathways (13).

SUMMARY

The 2-DG method of Sokoloff and colleagues (19) has proved valuable in identifying the neural substrates of reinforcement in the brain. A comparison of the patterns of cerebral metabolic activity activated by ICSS to the VTA and to the SN has isolated a reinforcement circuit that includes the medial prefrontal cortex, the nucleus accumbens, the lateral septum, and the mediodorsal nucleus of the thalamus. Activity within this circuit has also been shown to be specific to reinforced behavior and not merely a function of electrical stimulation alone. The use of this method in other paradigms in which behavior is reinforced by other types of reinforcers, e.g., drugs of abuse or natural reinforcers such as food, will provide further information about the nature of reward systems in the brain.

ACKNOWLEDGMENTS

Many thanks to my collaborators in this work, Dr. Ralph Esposito, Dr. Thomas Seeger, Dr. Agu Pert, and Alison Crane. Special thanks to Dr. Louis Sokoloff for collaboration, encouragement, and support in the conduct of these studies, as well as his comments on the manuscript. The editorial assistance of Brenda Sandler is also gratefully acknowledged.

REFERENCES

1. Beckstead, R. M., Domesick, V. B., and Nauta, W. J. (1979): Efferent connections of the substantia nigra and ventral tegmental area in the rat. *Brain Res.,* 175:191–217.

2. Crow, T. J. (1972): A map of the rat mesencephalon for electrical self-stimulation. *Brain Res.,* 36:265–273.
3. Esposito, R. U., Porrino, L. J., Seeger, T. F., Crane, A. M., Everist, H. D., and Pert, A. (1984): Changes in local cerebral glucose utilization during rewarding brain stimulation. *Proc. Natl. Acad. Sci. USA,* 81:635–639.
4. Gallistel, C. R., Karreman, G. A., and Reivich, M. (1977): [^{14}C]-2-deoxyglucose uptake marks systems activated by rewarding brain stimulation. *Brain Res. Bull.,* 2:149–152.
5. Olds, J., and Milner, P. (1954): Positive reinforcement produced by electrical stimulation of septal area and other regions of rat brain. *Journal of Comparative and Physiological Psychology,* 47:419–427.
6. Olds, M. E., and Fobes, J. L. (1981): The central basis of motivation: Intracranial self-stimulation studies. *Annu. Rev. Psychol.,* 32:523–574.
7. Phillips, A. G., LePiane, F. G., and Fibiger, H. C. (1982): Effects of kainic acid lesions of the striatum on self-stimulation in the substantia nigra and ventral tegmental area. *Behav. Brain Res.,* 5:297–310.
8. Porrino, L. J., Esposito, R. U., Seeger, T., and Crane, A. M. (1985): Patterns of brain energy metabolism associated with rewarding brain stimulation of the substantia nigra. *J. Cereb. Blood Flow Metab.,* 5 (Suppl. 1):S211–S212.
9. Porrino, L. J., Esposito, R. U., Seeger, T. F., Crane, A. M., Jehle, J. W., Sullivan, T., Pert, A., and Sokoloff, L. (1984): A comparison of self-stimulation to the ventral tegmental area and substantia nigra in the rat by means of 2-[^{14}C]deoxyglucose autoradiography. *Society for Neuroscience Abstracts,* 10:307.
10. Porrino, L. J., Esposito, R. U., Seeger, T. F., Crane, A. M., Pert, A., and Sokoloff, L. (1984): Metabolic mapping of brain during rewarding self-stimulation. *Science,* 224:306–309.
11. Porrino, L. J., and Lucignani, G. (1986): Different patterns of brain energy metabolism associated with high and low doses of methylphenidate: Implications for stimulant drug action in hyperactive children (*in press*).
12. Porrino, L. J., Lucignani, G., Dow-Edwards, D., and Sokoloff, L. (1984): Dose-dependent effects of acute amphetamine administration on functional brain metabolism in rats. *Brain Res.,* 307: 311–320.
13. Seeger, T. F., Porrino, L. J., Esposito, R. U., Crane, A. M., Sullivan, T. L., and Pert, A. (1984): Amphetamine effects on intracranial self-stimulation as assessed by the quantitative 2-deoxyglucose method. *Society for Neuroscience Abstracts,* 10:307.
14. Skinner, B. F. (1938): *The Behavior of Organisms.* Appleton-Century Crofts, New York.
15. Smith, J. E., Co, C., Freeman, M. E., and Lane, J. D. (1982): Brain neurotransmitter turnover correlated with morphine-seeking behavior of rats. *Pharmacol. Biochem. Behav.,* 16:509–519.
16. Smith, J. E., Co, C., and Lane, J. D. (1984): Limbic acetylcholine turnover rates correlated with rat morphine-seeking behaviors. *Pharmacol. Biochem. Behav.,* 20:429–441.
17. Smith, J. E., Co, C., and Lane, J. D. (1984): Limbic muscarinic cholinergic and benzodiazepine receptor changes with chronic intravenous morphine and self-administration. *Pharmacol. Biochem. Behav.,* 20:443–450.
18. Sokoloff, L. (1982): The radioactive deoxyglucose method. Theory, procedure, and applications for the measurement of local glucose utilization in the central nervous system. In: *Advances in Neurochemistry, Vol. 4.,* edited by B. W. Agranoff and M. H. Aprison, pp. 1–82. Plenum Publishing Corp., New York.
19. Sokoloff, L., Reivich, M., Kennedy, C., Des Rosiers, M. H., Patlak, C. S., Pettigrew, K. D., Sakurada, O., and Shinohara, M. (1977): The [^{14}C]deoxyglucose method for the measurement of local cerebral glucose utilization: Theory, procedure, and normal values in the conscious and anesthetized albino rat. *J. Neurochem.,* 28:897–916.
20. Stein, L. (1962): Effects and interactions of imipramine, chlorpromazine, reserpine and amphetamine on self-stimulation: Possible neurophysiological basis of depression. In *Recent Advances in Biological Psychiatry, Vol. 4,* edited by J. Wortis, pp. 288–308. Plenum Press, New York.
21. Steiner, S. S., Beer, B., and Shaffer, M. M. (1968): Escape from self-produced rates of brain stimulation. *Science,* 163:90–91.
22. Trowill, J. A., Panksepp, J., and Gandelman, R. (1969): An incentive model of rewarding brain stimulation. *Psychol. Rev.,* 76:264–287.
23. Yadin, E., Guarini, V., and Gallistel, C. R. (1983): Unilaterally activated systems in rats self-stimulating at sites in the medial forebrain bundle, medial prefrontal cortex, or locus coeruleus. *Brain Res.,* 266:39–50.

Brain Reward Systems and Abuse, edited by
J. Engel and L. Oreland.
Raven Press, New York © 1987.

Role of Catecholamine Transmitters in Brain Reward Systems: Implications for the Neurobiology of Affect

H. C. Fibiger and *A. G. Phillips

*Division of Neurological Sciences, Departments of Psychiatry and *Psychology,
University of British Columbia, Vancouver, B.C., V6T 1W5, Canada*

The neurobiological substrates of reward have been an active and important subject of research since the classic experiments of Olds and Milner (30), who showed that an animal will work to stimulate electrically certain parts of its brain. A major goal in this area of research has been to map neural circuits that mediate the rewarding properties of brain stimulation, the assumption being that a thorough understanding of these circuits would provide a basis for studying reward circuits that are activated by natural reinforcers.

NORADRENALINE HYPOTHESIS

Early studies on brain stimulation reward (BSR) led to the proposal that noradrenergic (NA) projections originating in the locus ceruleus are an important substrate for BSR (7,12,48). This was based primarily on the findings that intracranial self-stimulation (ICSS) can be obtained from brain regions that are innervated by the locus ceruleus and that drugs that facilitate transmission at NA synapses enhance ICSS, while drugs that interfere with NA transmission have the opposite effect. The NA hypothesis of BSR received further indirect support with the discovery that tricyclic antidepressant drugs are potent NA-uptake inhibitors and thereby increase the synaptic concentrations of this neurotransmitter. It was hypothesized that the antidepressant properties of the tricyclic drugs may be related to their ability to enhance the function of this noradrenergic reward-related system, the activity of which may be abnormally low in depressed patients.

This seemingly satisfying state of affairs continued until the mid 1970s when a number of papers were published that cast serious doubt on the NA hypothesis of reward. The details of the now large body of evidence that contradicts the predictions of the NA hypothesis have been reviewed previously and need not be reiterated here (9,51). Suffice it to say that in retrospect the pharmacological evidence for the NA hypothesis was weak both in terms of the specificity of the drugs that were used and in terms of the use of behavioral methodologies that often failed to adequately control for nonreward-related effects of the drugs. Perhaps more importantly, the introduction of 6-hydroxydopamine (6-OHDA) made it possible to produce extensive and selective lesions of the NA systems and to study the effects of these lesions on ICSS. In contrast to the predictions of the NA hypothesis of reward, these lesions invariably failed to disrupt ICSS (9,51).

The circumstantial evidence provided by the proposed mechanism of action of tricyclic antidepressants (TCAs) was also superseded by new data inconsistent with the NA hypothesis. Specifically, while it is true that TCAs block the reuptake of synaptically released NA, it was subsequently discovered that chronic administration of these compounds leads to down-regulation of NA receptors on the postsynaptic neuron, a process that would offset TCA-induced increases in the synaptic availability of NA (see ref. 5 for review). The TCA-induced increase in synaptic concentrations of NA, coupled with the down-regulation of NA receptors, raises the question as to the net effect of chronic TCAs on adrenoceptive neurons. This can best be answered by neurophysiological experiments, and, although to date only a few studies have addressed this question, they indicate that the net effect of chronic administration of TCAs is to decrease the level of noradrenergic transmission in the CNS (16,17,31,49). From this perspective, if NA mechanisms play any role in the therapeutic actions of TCAs then it would have to be attributed to a decrease in the functional activity of the NA systems rather than by facilitating their function as originally proposed. On the basis of evidence such as this, it could be argued that the NA projections of the locus ceruleus are involved in the processing of aversive stimuli, including perhaps emotional reactions to punishment or loss of reward. In this regard, it is noteworthy that many aversive stimuli including footshock, cold, and restraint stress reliably increase the activity of the locus ceruleus (1). Also, 6-OHDA lesions of the dorsal NA bundle, through which courses the major NA innervation of the telencephalon, greatly attenuate the aversive effects of morphine as measured by the conditioned taste aversion procedure (38). These considerations raise the possibility that the activity of the locus ceruleus is excessive in some forms of depression and that TCAs produce their therapeutic actions by decreasing the influence of this noradrenergic system on neurons postsynaptic to it.

MESOLIMBIC DOPAMINE HYPOTHESIS

The demise of the NA reward hypothesis provided new impetus for identifying alternate neural mechanisms by which indirectly acting sympathomimetics such as amphetamine and cocaine enhance ICSS. Although early work emphasized the NA actions of these drugs, it has long been known that these compounds also have potent actions on the release and/or reuptake of dopamine (DA) by central DA neurons. This raised the possibility that certain DA projections are themselves important substrates for BSR or that DA systems somehow facilitate the function of nonDA reward-related systems. The result of a considerable body of research over the past decade indicated that the mesolimbic DA projection is itself an important reward-related system. We will review some of the data that have led to this conclusion. Additional pertinent data are contained in the chapters by M. A. Bozarth and by G. F. Koob et al. (*this volume*).

The mesolimbic DA projection arises primarily from neurons in the ventral tegmental area (VTA). By definition these neurons innervate limbic regions such as the nucleus accumbens, lateral septum, olfactory tubercle, and amygdala. Very high and stable rates of ICSS can be obtained from the VTA. Although this would be consistent with an important role for mesolimbic DA neurons in reward, additional studies are required to show that DA neurons, as opposed to nonDA elements in the VTA, mediate some of the rewarding effects of ICSS obtained from this region.

The results of the first such study were reported by Phillips and Fibiger (33), who found that 6-OHDA lesions of the ascending fibers of the mesotelencephalic DA projection resulted in marked decreases in rates of responding for ICSS obtained from electrodes in the VTA. Self-stimulation obtained from electrodes in the frontal cortex or nucleus accumbens of the same animals was not as severely affected suggesting that the marked effects on VTA-ICSS could not be attributed entirely to lesion-induced motor deficits. Subsequent work in our laboratories has confirmed and extended these findings. Rats were again trained to self-stimulate from electrodes in the VTA. In addition, ICSS rate–current intensity functions were obtained. These functions determine the rate of responding for ICSS at various brain stimulation current intensities and provide more detailed information than can be obtained with single current intensities. After rate–intensity functions had been determined, the animals received 6-OHDA lesions of the mesotelencephalic DA projections at the level of the lateral hypothalamus. These lesions were either ipsilateral or contralateral to the ICSS electrode in the VTA.

The results of this experiment are presented in Fig. 1, where it can be seen that 6-OHDA lesions ipsilateral to the ICSS electrode produced a marked shift to the right in the rate–intensity function. In contrast, identical lesions contralateral to the electrode failed to produce significant shifts in the rate–intensity function. These results indicate that the lesions did not produce significant motor deficits and that the decreases in ICSS produced by the ipsilateral lesions were likely due to a decrease in the rewarding properties of the brain stimulation. In animals with ipsilateral 6-OHDA lesions, it was possible to reinstate some ICSS at the higher current intensities (Fig. 1). This may have been mediated by the few DA neurons that survived the 6-OHDA lesions or by nonDA elements in the VTA that were capable of supporting a degree of brain stimulation reward.

Pharmacological studies also point to an important role for the mesolimbic DA system in the rewarding properties of ICSS obtained from the VTA. In what

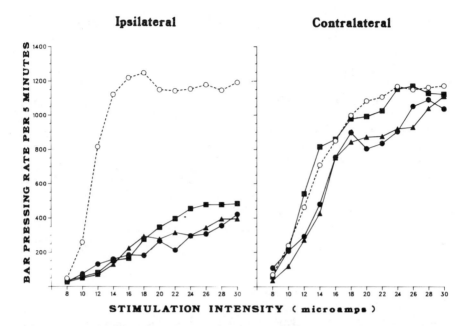

FIG. 1. The effect of extensive (>90% DA depletion) 6-OHDA lesions of the mesotelencephalic DA projections on ICSS obtained from electrodes in the VTA. The lesions were either ipsilateral or contralateral to the ICSS electrode. Note the marked effects of ipsilateral lesions on the ICSS rate–current intensity functions and the failure of the contralateral lesions to affect these functions. The data represent the means of 8 (ipsilateral) and 7 (contralateral) animals. *Open circle,* pretest; *filled circle,* posttest 3; *filled square,* posttest 9; *filled triangle,* posttest 18.

is perhaps the definitive study on this question, Mogenson et al. (29) found that unilateral injections of the DA receptor antagonist spiroperidol into the nucleus accumbens significantly reduced ICSS of the ipsilateral VTA but did not affect the rate of ICSS obtained from the contralateral VTA. The contrasting effects of the ipsilateral and contralateral nucleus accumbens injections on VTA-ICSS indicate that spiroperidol-induced motor deficits cannot account for these observations. The specificity of the effect of the ipsilateral nucleus accumbens injections was also demonstrated by the finding that injections of spiroperidol into either the ipsilateral or contralateral prefrontal cortex did not affect VTA-ICSS. Therefore, in contrast to the nucleus accumbens, DA receptors in the prefrontal cortex do not appear to be important for mediating the rewarding effects of VTA-ICSS. As will be seen later, similar conclusions have been reached with respect to the rewarding properties of intravenously self-administered cocaine.

Further evidence that DA neurons are an important substrate for VTA-ICSS has been obtained in biochemical experiments. Simon et al. (44) first demonstrated that DA metabolism, as expressed by the ratio of the DA metabolite 3,4-dihydroxyphenylacetic acid (DOPAC) to DA was increased in the nucleus accumbens and frontal cortex of rats that self-stimulated through electrodes in the

VTA. These results have recently been confirmed and extended in our laboratories. In the latter experiments, VTA-ICSS increased both DOPAC/DA and homovanillic acid HVA/DA ratios in the striatum, nucleus accumbens, and olfactory tubercle, thus providing direct evidence that DA neurons are activated during ICSS in the VTA (Figs. 2 and 3). This activation was confined to the side of the brain ipsilateral to the stimulating electrode, indicating that the increased DA utilization was due to the electrical stimulation rather than the high level of operant behavior displayed by the animal during the ICSS sessions. This conclusion has received further endorsement from the observation of increased concentrations of DOPA in these same regions after VTA-ICSS in rats pretreated with the DOPA decarboxylase inhibitor NSD-1015 (Fig. 4). Again these biochemical changes were only seen in the hemisphere ipsilateral to the VTA stimulating electrode.

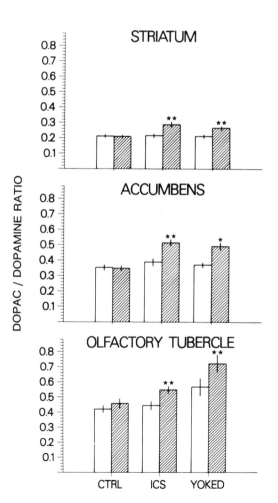

FIG. 2. The effects of ICSS obtained from electrodes in the VTA on DOPAC/DA ratios in three dopamine-rich forebrain regions. Control animals (ctrl; $N = 12$) were implanted with electrodes but received no brain stimulation. The ICS group ($N = 9$) were killed immediately after 30 min of self-stimulation. Animals in the yoked group ($N = 4$) received brain stimulation at the same current and rate as matched animals in the ICS group but did not control the delivery of the brain stimulation and were killed after 30 min of the imposed brain stimulation. Dopamine and DOPAC were measured by HPLC. Note the increase in the DOPAC/DA ratios in all three forebrain regions on the side ipsilateral to the electrode in the ICS and yoked groups. *$p < 0.05$; **$p < 0.01$; compared to the contralateral side. Open bar, contralateral; shaded bar, ipsilateral.

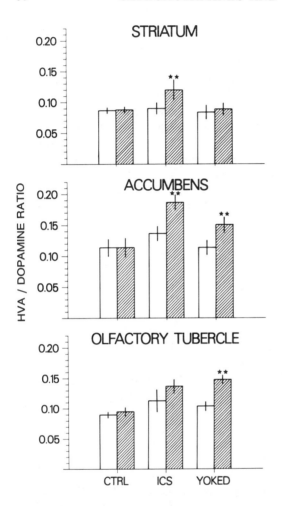

FIG. 3. The effects of ICSS obtained from electrodes in the VTA on HVA/DA ratios in three dopamine-rich forebrain regions. See Fig. 2 for details. **$p < 0.01$ compared to contralateral side. *Open bar,* contralateral; *shaded bar,* ipsilateral.

The demonstration that DA neurons are clearly stimulated during VTA-ICSS and that VTA-ICSS is severely disrupted by 6-OHDA lesions of the mesotelencephalic DA projections provides strong evidence that these neurons are an important neural substrate for ICSS obtained from this part of the brain. Other evidence indicating that the mesolimbic DA projection is a reward-related system has been obtained from studies of intravenous drug self-administration. Since the classic work of Weeks (50), it has been known that animals will work to deliver intravenous injections of various classes of psychoactive drugs, including stimulants and narcotics. Several studies suggest that the reinforcing properties of stimulants such as cocaine and *d*-amphetamine are mediated by the effects of these compounds on DA release in the nucleus accumbens. In the first of these studies, Roberts et al. (37) trained rats to self-administer cocaine. After stable daily response rates had been achieved, the animals received bilateral

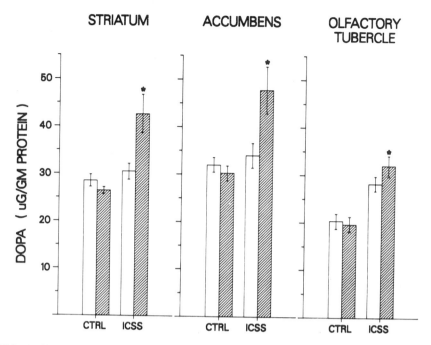

FIG. 4. The effect of ICSS obtained from the VTA on the accumulation of DOPA in brain regions ipsilateral or contralateral to the electrode after injections of the DOPA decarboxylase inhibitor NSD-1015 (50 mg/kg, i.p.). The drug was injected 5 min prior to a 30-min self-stimulation session (ICSS group) after which the animals were immediately killed. Control animals (CTRL) were implanted with VTA electrodes. They received NSD-1015 but were not given the opportunity to self-stimulate on the test day. Regional concentrations of DOPA were measured by HPLC. Note the increase in *in vivo* tyrosine hydroxylase activity (as measured by the accumulation of DOPA) in all three brain regions ipsilateral to the VTA electrode in the ICSS group. Data represent means (±SEM) of 6 animals in each group. *$p < 0.05$, compared to contralateral side. *Open bar*, contralateral; *shaded bar*, ipsilateral.

6-OHDA lesions of the nucleus accumbens. It was found that animals with extensive losses of DA in the nucleus accumbens showed large decreases in the rate at which they lever-pressed for intravenous injections of cocaine. It is noteworthy that 6-OHDA lesions of the dorsal and ventral NA bundles, which caused large and widespread decreases in the concentration of NA in the forebrain, had no effect on the rate or pattern of cocaine self-administration. It appears, therefore, that central NA systems do not contribute significantly either to electrical brain stimulation or to stimulant-induced reward. In another study, Lyness et al. (23) found similar effects of 6-OHDA lesions of the nucleus accumbens on *d*-amphetamine self-administration.

Roberts et al. (39) analyzed the pattern of self-administration of cocaine after 6-OHDA lesions of the nucleus accumbens. On the first day after the 6-OHDA lesions that they were given access to cocaine, the animals responded rapidly for the drug early in the 3-hr session. However, as the session progressed, the rate of responding decreased gradually until there was little or no responding by the end of the session. Similar patterns were found on the following few days except that early responding was reduced and cessation of responding occurred more quickly. These data are presented in Fig. 5 and are important for several reasons. First, the high rate of responding for cocaine early in the first postlesion session indicated that the effects of the 6-OHDA lesions on cocaine self-administration could not be attributed to lesion-induced motor deficits. The fact that the lesions did not affect responding for the directly acting DA agonist apomorphine was

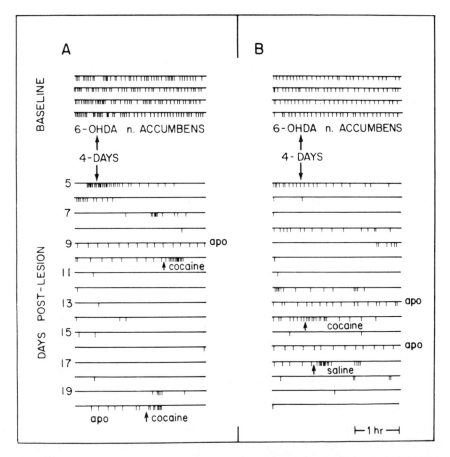

FIG. 5. Event records of cocaine self-administration after 6-OHDA infusions into the nucleus accumbens. Each line represents one daily 3-hr session. Downward pen deflections indicate drug injections. **A:** Example of cessation of responding for cocaine 5 days after 6-OHDA treatment. On postlesion day 9, regular responding is evident for apomorphine. On days 10 and 20, cocaine was substituted for apomorphine, which produced an initial burst of responding followed by cessation. **B:** Another example of extinction of cocaine self-administration 5 days after 6-OHDA treatment. Apomorphine self-administration is shown on days 13, 14, 16, and 17. Cocaine and saline were substituted for apomorphine on days 14 and 17 respectively. (From Roberts et al., ref. 39, with permission.)

consistent with this interpretation. Second, the pattern of cocaine self-administration after the 6-OHDA lesions resembled a classic extinction effect. Typically this has been characterized by high rates of responding when a reinforcer is first removed, which is followed by gradually decreasing rates of responding as the animal learns that the operant response no longer results in the delivery of a reward. The most parsimonious interpretation of this pattern of results is that extensive 6-OHDA lesions of the nucleus accumbens block the reinforcing effects of intravenous cocaine.

The data reviewed above suggest that DA terminals in the nucleus accumbens or a DA projection coursing through it are necessary for the normal expression of amphetamine and cocaine reinforcement. Martin-Iverson et al. (25) have recently addressed the possibility that some of the effect of 6-OHDA lesions of the nucleus accumbens on cocaine self-administration is due to damage of mesocortical DA axons that pass through this nucleus. This gained importance with the report by Goeders and Smith (13) that rats would not self-administer cocaine directly into the nucleus accumbens but would initiate and maintain responding for cocaine when infusion cannulae were placed in the medial prefrontal cortex. Martin-Iverson et al. (25) trained rats to self-administer cocaine intravenously, and when stable rates of responding were obtained, bilateral 6-OHDA lesions were aimed at the medial prefrontal cortex. It was found that the lesions failed to affect either the rate or pattern of cocaine self-administration, although substantial decreases in the concentration of DA in the medial prefrontal cortex were observed. These results suggest that DA terminals in the medial prefrontal cortex are not a critical substrate for the rewarding properties of intravenous cocaine. Although the basis of the discrepancy between these results and those of Goeders and Smith (13) is not readily apparent, it is possible that intracerebral self-administration of cocaine is related more to its local anesthetic properties than to its effects on DA uptake. In any event, the results of Martin-Iverson et al. (25) are congruent with data of Mogenson et al. (29) who, it will be recalled, found that injection of spiroperidol into the nucleus accumbens but not in the prefrontal cortex reduced ICSS obtained from electrodes in the VTA.

The finding that the meso–accumbens DA projection is a link in a reward-related circuit raises a number of interesting questions. For example, are there reward circuits that do not contain this DA link or is the meso–accumbens DA projection a common link in all such circuits, as has been proposed by Wise (52)? What are the natural stimuli in the environment that increase the activity of the system? According to Wise (52), all rewarding stimuli should activate this system. Do they? The fact that subhedonia or anhedonia is an invariant feature of clinical depression raises the question of whether this results from a pathologically low level of activity in the meso–accumbens DA projection in some forms of depression. Is it possible that some antidepressant drugs produce their beneficial effects by restoring the normal activity of this reward-related DA system? If so, by what mechanisms might this occur? Data that are pertinent to some of these issues are reviewed below.

DOPAMINE-INDEPENDENT REWARD CIRCUITS

As noted above, Wise (52) has proposed that part of the mesotelencephalic DA projection, probably the mesolimbic component, may be a final common reward pathway in the CNS. Current evidence indicates that this is not the case. One prediction of this hypothesis is that all electrodes that support ICSS, regardless of their location in the brain, should either directly or indirectly activate this DA system. This has been refuted by Mitchell et al. (28) who demonstrated that although DA turnover can be increased by ICSS obtained from electrodes in the VTA, this does not occur during stimulation of other sites from which equally high rates of ICSS can be obtained. Wise's (52) hypothesis also predicts that administration of DA receptor antagonists should block or blunt the effects of all rewarding stimuli and be similar to putting an animal into a state of non-reinforcement, i.e., extinction. Although similarities between the effects of neuroleptics and nonreward have been demonstrated in some situations, important differences have been observed between neuroleptic administration and extinction in a variety of other circumstances (2,15,26,34,52). Also, although the rewarding effects of intravenous cocaine can be blocked by 6-OHDA lesions of the nucleus accumbens, these lesions have no effect on operant responding for food, suggesting that the rewarding properties of food are not strongly dependent on DA release in the nucleus accumbens (37). Similarly, heroin-induced reward does not appear to have the same critical dependency on DA terminals in the nucleus accumbens as does cocaine-induced reward (32). None of these findings are easily accommodated by Wise's (52) hypothesis.

Recent experiments by Gallistel et al. (11) using 2-deoxy-D-[^{14}C]glucose autoradiography have shown that it is possible to obtain relatively high rates of ICSS from electrodes in the posterior hypothalamus without metabolic activation in terminal regions of the mesotelencephalic DA systems. However, the brain stimulation significantly increased metabolic activity in other brain regions, suggesting that separate systems can subserve brain stimulation reward and that these systems can function independently of the mesolimbic DA system. Thus, the mesolimbic DA reward system and the nonDA systems studied by Gallistel et al. (11) appear to function in parallel rather than being connected in series as would be predicted by Wise's (52) hypothesis. On the basis of these considerations, it can be concluded that the meso–accumbens DA projection is one link in a reward-related system and that there exist other reward circuits that do not contain this DA link.

Although enhanced DA release from terminals of the mesolimbic system, be it produced by electrical stimulation or by stimulant drugs, is sufficient to produce reward, at present the identity of naturally occurring stimuli that increase or decrease the activity of this system remains largely unknown. Neuroleptics can block the establishment of conditioned reinforcement when food is used as a primary reinforcer (4,47). Also, using a behavioral contrast procedure, Royall and Klemm (40) have obtained data which suggest that in rats the perceived rewarding value of a saccharin solution is decreased by haloperidol. It still remains to be determined whether neuroleptics impair the function of a DA system activated directly by the primary rewarding stimuli associated with food and saccharin or whether they impair DA mechanisms that mediate subsequent reactions to reward-related stimuli, as implied by the concept of incentive motivation. It can be anticipated that the application of techniques such as *in vivo* voltammetry and brain dialysis in behaving animals will answer many of these important questions.

CLINICAL IMPLICATIONS: A DOPAMINE–ACETYLCHOLINE BALANCE IN THE CONTROL OF AFFECT

An impaired ability to experience pleasure or reward (i.e., anhedonia) is invariably associated with clinical depression. The fact that the meso–accumbens DA projection is a reward-related system raises the possibility that dysfunction of this system may either be the cause of or contribute to some forms of depression. It also raises the possibility that some antidepressant treatments may produce their therapeutic effects by enhancing the function of this reward-related DA system. Evidence from a number of laboratories is compatible with this hypothesis. For example, a variety of procedures that are known to be useful in the treatment of depression have been shown to enhance the function of central DA systems. This includes chronic administration of TCAs (6,42,46), electroconvulsive shock (3,14,41), and rapid eye movement sleep deprivation (43). Fibiger and Phillips (10) found that ICSS obtained from electrodes in the VTA was enhanced by chronic but not acute administration of desipramine. In addition, chronic administration of some antidepressant drugs increases the locomotor stimulant response to *d*-amphetamine (24,46), a response that has previously been shown to be mediated by the meso–accumbens DA projection (21,22).

Although the mechanism by which these antidepressant drugs enhance the function of the meso–accumbens DA projection is not currently known, Martin-Iverson et al. (24) have proposed that their anticholinergic properties may be responsible for this effect and, by extension, may contribute to their antidepressant properties. In neurology, it has long been known that there exists a functional balance between dopaminergic and cholinergic mechanisms in the extrapyramidal system (27). Perhaps a similar balance exists in the neural circuitry that mediates affective processes and where excessive shifts in the direction of cholinergic (muscarinic) function are associated with depression, whereas abnormally enhanced dopaminergic tone is associated with mania. In humans, cocaine and amphetamine produce effects that resemble mania, whereas dopamine receptor antagonists are effective in the treatment of idiopathic manic states. On the cholinergic side, there is evidence for increased central cholinergic tone in depressed patients (35,45). Intravenous administration of the cholinesterase inhibitor physostigmine causes depressive effects on mood (36), leads to slowed thoughts, and decreases speech and spontaneous behavior (8). Also, physostig-mine diminishes manic symptomatology (19).

These findings, together with the ability of some antidepressants to enhance the function of the meso–accumbens DA reward system, are consistent with the hypothesis that the anticholinergic properties of some antidepressant drugs may contribute to their therapeutic effects. In this regard, it is interesting that there are numerous anecdotal reports that anticholinergic drugs have antidepressant effects (see ref. 18), and, in a controlled study, Kasper et al. (20) found that the anticholinergic drug biperidin was effective in the treatment of depression.

The evidence briefly reviewed above is consistent with the hypothesis that meso–accumbens DA neurons and presently unspecified cholinergic neurons are two components in the neural circuitry of affect. Disturbances in a functional balance between these two systems can lead to disturbances in affect—mania being associated with hyperdopaminergic tone and depression with hyperchol-inergic (muscarinic) function. A corollary of this hypothesis is that the therapeutic effects of some antidepressant drugs may be related to their antimuscarinic ac-tions. It is important to recognize, however, that not all antidepressants have significant anticholinergic properties. These drugs, therefore, must produce their clinically beneficial actions through other mechanisms. Given the complexity of the neural substrates of affect, this is not surprising. Apart from the dopa-minergic and cholinergic synapses, there are undoubtedly many other points at which the overall function of this circuitry can be influenced. The chemical identification of these other synapses is an important priority for future research, because it could lead to a new pharmacology of affective illness.

ACKNOWLEDGMENTS

Original findings contained in this manuscript were obtained with the support of the Medical Research Council of Canada (Program Grant 23). The excellent assistance of A. Jakubovic, F. Le Piane, D. Lin, and S. Atmadja is gratefully acknowledged.

REFERENCES

1. Anisman, H. (1978): Neurochemical changes elicited by stress. In: *Psychopharmacology of Aver-sively Motivated Behavior,* edited by H. Anisman and G. Bignami, pp. 119–172. Plenum Publishing Corporation, New York.
2. Asin, K. E., and Fibiger, H. C. (1984): Force requirements in lever-pressing and responding after haloperidol. *Pharmacol. Biochem. Behav.,* 20:323–326.
3. Balldin, J., Granerus, A. K., Lindstedt, G., Modish, K., and Walinder, J. (1982): Neuroendocrine evidence for increased responsiveness of dopamine receptors in humans following electroconvulsive therapy. *Psychopharmacology (Berlin),* 76:371–376.
4. Beninger, R. J., and Phillips, A. G. (1980): The effect of pimozide on the establishment of conditioned reinforcement. *Psychopharmacology (Berlin),* 68:147–153.
5. Charney, D. S., Menkes, D. B., and Heninger, G. R. (1981): Receptor sensitivity and the mech-anism of action of antidepressant treatment. *Arch. Gen. Psychiatry,* 38:1160–1180.

6. Chiodo, L. A., and Antelman, S. M. (1980): Tricyclic antidepressants induce subsensitivity of presynaptic dopamine autoreceptors. *Eur. J. Pharmacol.,* 64:203–204.
7. Crow, T. J. (1972): Catecholamine-containing neurones and electrical self-stimulation. 1. A review of some data. *Psychol. Med.,* 2:414–421.
8. Davis, K. L., Hollister, L. E., Overall, J., Johnson, A., and Train, K. (1976): Physostigmine effects on cognitive and affect in normal subjects. *Psychopharmacologia,* 51:23–29.
9. Fibiger, H. C. (1978): Drugs and reinforcement mechanisms: A critical review of the catecholamine theory. *Ann. Rev. Pharmacol. Toxicol.,* 18:37–56.
10. Fibiger, H. C., and Phillips, A. G. (1981): Increased intracranial self-stimulation in rats after long-term administration of desipramine. *Science,* 214:683–685.
11. Gallistel, C. R., Gomita, Y., Yadin, E., and Campbell, K. A. (1985): Forebrain origins and terminations of the medial forebrain bundle metabolically activated by rewarding stimulation or by reward-blocking doses of pimozide. *J. Neurosci.,* 5:1246–1261.
12. German, D. C., and Bowden, D. M. (1974): Catecholamine systems at the neural substrate for intracranial self-stimulation: A hypothesis. *Brain Res.,* 73:381–419.
13. Goeders, N. E., and Smith, J. E. (1983): Cortical involvement in cocaine reinforcement. *Science,* 221:773–775.
14. Green, A. R., and Deakin, J. F. W. (1980): Brain noradrenaline depletion prevents ECS-induced enhancement of serotonin- and dopamine-mediated behavior. *Nature,* 285:232–233.
15. Greenshaw, A. J., Sanger, D. J., and Blackman, D. E. (1981): The effects of pimozide and of reward omission on fixed-interval behavior of rats maintained by food and electrical brain stimulation. *Pharmacol. Biochem. Behav.,* 15:227–233.
16. Huang, Y. H. (1979): Chronic desipramine treatment increases activity of noradrenergic postsynaptic cells. *Life Sci.,* 25:709–716.
17. Huang, Y. H., Maas, J. W., and Hu, G. H. (1980): The time course of noradrenergic pre- and postsynaptic activity during chronic desipramine treatment. *Eur. J. Pharmacol.,* 68:41–47.
18. Janowsky, D. S., El-Yousef, M. K., Davis, J. M., and Sekerke, H. J. (1972): A cholinergic-adrenergic hypothesis of mania and depression. *Lancet,* 2:632–635.
19. Janowsky, D. S., El-Yousef, M. K., Davis, J. M., and Sekerke, H. J. (1973): Parasympathetic suppression of manic symptoms by physostigmine. *Arch. Gen. Psychiatry,* 28:542–547.
20. Kasper, S., Moises, H. W., and Beckman, H. (1981): The anticholinergic biperidin in depressive disorders. *Pharmacopsychiatry,* 14:195–198.
21. Kelly, P. H., and Iversen, S. D. (1976): Selective 6-OHDA induced destruction of mesolimbic dopamine neurons: Abolition of psychostimulant induced locomotor activity in rats. *Eur. J. Pharmacol.,* 40:45–56.
22. Koob, G. F., Stinus, L., and LeMoal, M. (1981): Hyperactivity and hypoactivity produced by lesions to the mesolimbic dopamine system. *Behav. Brain Res.,* 3:341–359.
23. Lyness, W. H., Friedle, N. M., and Moore, K. E. (1979): Destruction of dopaminergic nerve terminals in nucleus accumbens: Effect on d-amphetamine self-administration. *Pharmacol. Biochem. Behav.,* 11:553–556.
24. Martin-Iverson, M. T., Leclere, J. F., and Fibiger, H. C. (1983): Cholinergic-dopaminergic interactions and the mechanisms of action of antidepressants. *Eur. J. Pharmacol.,* 94:193–201.
25. Martin-Iverson, M. T., Szostak, C., and Fibiger, H. C. (1986): 6-Hydroxydopamine lesions of the medial prefrontal cortex fail to influence intravenous self-administration of cocaine. *Psychopharmacology (Berlin),* 88:310–314.
26. Mason, S. T., Beninger, R. J., Fibiger, H. C., and Phillips, A. G. (1980): Pimozide-induced suppression of responding: Evidence against a block of food reward. *Pharmacol. Biochem. Behav.,* 12:917–923.
27. McGeer, P. L., Boulding, J. E., Gibson, W. C., and Foulkes, R. G. (1961): Drug-induced extrapyramidal reactions: Treatment with diphenhydramine hydrochloride and dihydroxyphenylalanine. *J. A. M. A.,* 177:665–670.
28. Mitchell, M. J., Nicolaou, N. M., Arbuthnott, G. W., and Yates, C. M. (1982): Increases in dopamine metabolism are not a general feature of intracranial self-stimulation. *Life Sci.,* 30:1081–1085.
29. Mogenson, G. J., Takigawa, M., Robertson, A., and Wu, M. (1979): Self-stimulation of the nucleus accumbens and ventral tegmental area of Tsai attenuated by microinjections of spiroperidol into the nucleus accumbens. *Brain Res.,* 171:247–259.
30. Olds, J., and Milner, P. (1954): Positive reinforcement produced by electrical stimulation of septal area and other regions of rat brain. *Journal of Comparative and Physiological Psychology,* 47:419–427.

31. Olpe, H. R., and Schellenberg, A. (1980): Reduced sensitivity of neurons to noradrenaline after chronic treatment with antidepressant drugs. *Eur. J. Pharmacol.,* 63:7–13.

32. Pettit, H. O., Ettenberg, A., Bloom, F. E., and Koob, G. F. (1984): Destruction of dopamine in the nucleus accumbens selectively attenuates cocaine but not heroin self-administration in rats. *Psychopharmacology (Berlin),* 84:167–173.

33. Phillips, A. G., and Fibiger, H. C. (1978): The role of dopamine in maintaining intracranial self-stimulation in the ventral tegmentum, nucleus accumbens, medial and sulcal prefrontal cortices. *Can. J. Psychol.,* 32:58–66.

34. Phillips, A. G., and Fibiger, H. C. (1979): Decreased resistance to extinction after haloperidol: Implications for the role of dopamine in reinforcement. *Pharmacol. Biochem. Behav.,* 10:751–760.

35. Risch, S. C. (1982): β-Endorphin hypersecretion in depression: Possible cholinergic mechanisms. *Biol. Psychiatry,* 17:1071–1079.

36. Risch, S. C., Cohen, R. M., Janowsky, D. S., Kalin, N. H., and Murphy, D. L. (1980): Mood and behavioral effects of physostigmine on humans are accompanied by elevation in plasma β-endorphin and cortisol. *Science,* 209:1545–1546.

37. Roberts, D. C. S., Corcoran, M. E., and Fibiger, H. C. (1977): On the role of ascending catecholaminergic systems in intravenous self-administration of cocaine. *Pharmacol. Biochem. Behav.,* 6:615–620.

38. Roberts, D. C. S., and Fibiger, H. C. (1977): Lesions of the dorsal noradrenergic projection attenuate morphine but not amphetamine-induced conditioned taste aversion. *Psychopharmacology (Berlin),* 55:183–186.

39. Roberts, D. C. S., Koob, G. F., Klonoff, P., and Fibiger, H. C. (1980): Extinction and recovery of cocaine self-administration following 6-hydroxydopamine lesions of the nucleus accumbens. *Pharmacol. Biochem. Behav.,* 12:781–787.

40. Royall, D. R., and Klemm, W. R. (1981): Dopaminergic mediation of reward: Evidence gained using a natural reinforcer in a behavioral contrast paradigm. *Neurosci. Lett.,* 21:223–230.

41. Serra, G., Argiolas, A., Fadda, F., Melis, M. R., and Gessa, G. L. (1981): Repeated electroconvulsive shock prevents the sedative effect of small doses of apomorphine. *Psychopharmacology (Berlin),* 73:194–196.

42. Serra, G., Argiolas, A., Klimek, V., Fadda, F., and Gessa, G. L. (1979): Chronic treatment with antidepressants prevents the inhibitory effect of small doses of apomorphine on dopamine synthesis and motor activity. *Life Sci.,* 25:415–424.

43. Serra, G., Melis, M. R., Argiolas, A., Fadda, F., and Gessa, G. L. (1981): REM sleep deprivation induces subsensitivity of dopamine receptors mediating sedation in rats. *Eur. J. Pharmacol.,* 72:131–135.

44. Simon, H., Stinus, L., Tassin, J. P., Lavielle, S., Blanc, G., Thierry, A. M., Glowinski, J., and Le Moal, M. (1979): Is the dopaminergic mesocorticolimbic system necessary for intracranial self-stimulation? *Behav. Neurol Biol.,* 27:125–145.

45. Sitaram, N., Nurnberger, J. I., Gershon, E. S., and Gillin, J. C. (1980): Faster cholinergic REM sleep induction in euthymic patients with primary affective illness. *Science,* 208:200–202.

46. Spyraki, C., and Fibiger, H. C. (1981): Behavioral evidence for supersensitivity of postsynaptic dopamine receptors in the mesolimbic system after chronic administration of desipramine. *Eur. J. Pharmacol.,* 74:195–206.

47. Spyraki, C., Fibiger, H. C., and Phillips, A. G. (1982): Attenuation by haloperidol of place preference conditioning using food reinforcement. *Psychopharmacology (Berlin),* 77:379–382.

48. Stein, L., Belluzi, J. D., and Wise, C. D. (1976): Norepinephrine self-stimulation pathways: Implications for long-term memory and schizophrenia. In: *Brain–Stimulation Reward,* edited by A. Wauquier and E. T. Rolls, pp. 297–331. North-Holland Publishing, Amsterdam.

49. Svensson, T. H., and Usdin, T. (1978): Feedback inhibition of brain noradrenaline neurons by tricyclic antidepressants: Alpha-receptor mediation. *Science,* 202:1089–1091.

50. Weeks, J. R. (1962): Experimental morphine addiction: Method for automatic intravenous injections in unrestrained rats. *Science,* 138:143–144.

51. Wise, R. A. (1978): Catecholamine theories of reward: A critical review. *Brain Res.,* 152:215–247.

52. Wise, R. A. (1982): Neuroleptics and operant behaviour: The anhedonia hypothesis. *Behav. Brain Sci.,* 5:39–53.

Brain Reward Systems and Abuse, edited by
J. Engel and L. Oreland.
Raven Press, New York © 1987.

Reward and Abuse: Opiates and Neuropeptides

Jan M. Van Ree

Rudolf Magnus Institute for Pharmacology, Medical Faculty, University of Utrecht, 3521 GD Utrecht, The Netherlands

A variety of psychoactive drugs have been used for many centuries to influence the brain function of healthy individuals as well as of mentally disturbed patients. Some of these drugs are (self-)administered to such an extent that a state of drug dependence is achieved, which is characterized by the drug user performing substantial amounts of behavior leading specifically to further administration of the drug, even when this requires the sacrifice of other behaviors (34). Severe degrees of dependence are commonly labeled as addiction or abuse, particularly in clinical practice. Historically, studies on the addictive properties of drugs in experimental animals have mainly been focused on morphinomimetics and ethanol. These drugs also induce physical dependence, characterized by a specific pattern of biological events that occur in response to withdrawal of the drug. Although physical dependence has been considered as one of the most important mechanisms underlying drug addiction, recent research has not substantiated this assumption, as will be discussed below.

The concepts of operant behavior as formulated by Skinner (54) have had important consequences for the experimental analysis of drug dependence. These concepts have yielded the identification of a number of positively reinforcing or rewarding stimuli, called positive reinforcers, as can be determined by an increase of behavior that immediately precedes the presentation of the reinforcing stimulus. By performing that behavior, the organism increases the change of the reinforcing or rewarding stimulus to occur. For the present survey, the terms "reward" and "reinforcement" will be used interchangeably. An experimental situation in which the subject is given the opportunity to take a drug has been called self-administration. A number of models of drug self-administration have been developed during the last decades; one of the most frequently used is the intravenous self-administration in rats and monkeys (34). It has become increasingly clear that there are many drugs from various pharmacological classes that can serve as positive reinforcer in animal experiments (57,73). Thus, the occurrence of the behavioral pattern, which is followed by the administration of these drugs, is increased or maintained; the drugs are self-administered. Most of the drugs that initiate and maintain self-administering behavior in laboratory animals are abused to some extent in humans. Conversely, psychoactive drugs that fail to initiate and maintain self-administration are not readily abused by humans. Thus, empirically and theoretically the self-administration technique is a useful method to predict the abuse potential of drugs (10). It establishes the reinforcing efficacy of drugs and is reliably applicable to evaluate the variables that interfere with drug-taking behavior (62). These variables include external factors, drug-induced changes in the organism, and internal factors. Two of these internal factors may be distinguished: first, the neuronal substrate affected by addictive drugs, which, when activated, produce reinforcement; and second, factors that modulate the drug-induced reinforcing activity. Both factors may be critical for the initiation of self-administration and may contribute to the individual susceptibility to addictive drugs with respect to drug-taking behavior. Candidates for these factors are the neuropeptides—endogenous molecules in which specific information is encoded. In the present survey, the significance of neuropeptides for opiate reward will be discussed.

OPIATE REWARD

Although the intravenous self-administration procedure is the most widely accepted method of assessing the reinforcing properties of abused drugs, other procedures have been proposed as well. These include the conditioned place preference, the intracranial self-administration, and the interaction with brain stimulation reward, which have also been applied with respect to opiates. In the conditioned place preference procedure, animals are tested under drug-free conditions to determine if a preference or aversion has developed to an environment that they have experienced before the effects of the drug. The intracranial self-administration procedure follows a similar method as the intravenous one, but the drug is infused directly into discrete brain regions, which may minimize the side effects caused by systemic drug injections. The intracranial electrical brain self-stimulation (ICSS) procedure is widely used to explore the significance of certain brain structures with respect to reward. Since there are several similarities between drug self-administration and ICSS behavior, it has been suggested that drugs are reinforcing because they interact with certain central reward structures that can also be activated by ICSS. The different variables that interfere with or are pertinent to opiate reward will be discussed. Especially data on the intravenous self-administration procedure will be mentioned, because the available information on the other procedures is limited in this respect.

Type of Drug

Morphine and related opiates have the ability to function as positive reinforcers. This was first suggested by Spragg (56), who showed that chimpanzees previously made physically dependent on morphine could learn to select of two boxes the one concealing a syringe filled with a morphine solution that would subsequently be administered to the animal by the experimenter. Self-injection by animals was first reported in 1955 by Headlee and co-workers (30), who demonstrated that morphine was injected intraperitoneally by physically dependent rats. Techniques for intravenous self-administration by both monkeys and rats were developed in the 1960s (14,50,80). With these techniques it was demonstrated that morphine and related opiates are self-administered by drug naive animals (14,74). A variety of opiate agonists, mixed agonists and antagonists, and antagonists have been studied as intravenous reinforcers. Opiate agonists, which exert morphine-like actions in other systems, have the capacity to function as positive reinforcers (82). A positive correlation between the potencies of such agonists in maintaining self-administration and in producing other morphine-like actions, e.g., analgesia and suppressing morphine abstinence, have been reported in both rats and monkeys (74,83). Opiate antagonists, like naloxone and naltrexone fail to maintain responding under conditions that are sufficient for self-administration of opiate agonists (82). Naloxone will even serve as a negative reinforcer (20). Opiates that can be characterized as mixed agonist-antagonists function as positive reinforcers but only when these drugs share agonist actions primarily with morphine-like opiates (82). Thus, the receptor systems mediating the reinforcing action of opiates seem similar to those mediating the other typical morphine-like actions of opiates.

External Factors

External factors affect the initiation, maintenance, and cessation of drug self-administration (34). These factors include the dose of the drug, the schedule and conditions of drug availability, and stimulus control among others. The dose of the drug is important for the observed ability of the drug to maintain self-administration. An intermediate dose range seems optimal for the initiation and maintenance of opiate self-administration, whereas very low and very high doses do not favor it. Thus, the rate of drug maintained responding is an inverted U-shaped function of dose (84). Varying the unit dose delivered per injection in the intermediate dose range during acquisition of opiate self-administration showed that increases in unit dose produce increases in total drug intake (74,78). Thus, the unit dose delivered is one of the factors that determine the ultimate level of drug intake, and the amount of drug taken can serve as a useful index of the reinforcing efficacy of the drug injection. Consistently, the extinction of opiate self-administering behavior is slower when the drug dose is higher, also suggesting that the reinforcing potential is increased when the unit dose increases (73). The schedule of drug availability has been studied during maintenance of drug self-administration, including with opiates. In general, the characteristics of the schedule-controlled behavior maintained by drug reinforcers cannot be distinguished from the characteristics of behaviors maintained by nondrug reinforcement (55). Drug self-administration is decreased when the response requirement and thus the amount of work that subjects have to expend to earn drug reinforcement increases. Higher doses of the drug are needed to maintain self-administration when the response requirement is higher and when the interinjection interval increases (32,84). During maintenance of drug self-administration, a variety of initially neutral environmental stimuli may influence the amount and pattern of drug-taking behavior. Among these are conditioned stimuli, which substantially increase the amount of drug intake and discriminative stimuli, that signal the occasion that drug reinforcement is available (29). Other environmental factors, e.g., social conditions, aversive conditions and the presence of nondrug reinforcers, will certainly interact with drug-seeking behavior, but information in this respect is limited.

Drug-Induced Changes in the Organism

The self-administered drug may alter a variety of homeostatic mechanisms in the body. These changes may contribute more or less to the behavior associated with drug-taking and alter the reinforcing properties of the drug. They include alterations in mood, e.g., euphoria and dysphoria, and in sexual, social, and aggressive behaviors (38). These subjective and objective effects elicited by the drug may themselves reinforce the drug-seeking behavior. The discriminative stimulus properties of drugs have been proposed as a model for the subjective effects of drugs (11). The test procedure involves the request that subjects evaluate the ability of the drug tested to produce subjective effects similar to those induced by the presently or formerly taken drug. It has extensively been shown that opiates can act as discriminative stimuli (13,52). This discriminative stimulus complex appears to be exclusively associated with the specific central actions of narcotic analgesic drugs, as may also hold for the reinforcing properties of opiates.

Also, the adaptive changes in the organism in response to repeated administration of opiates may be important for the drug-seeking behavior. These changes include the development of tolerance and physical dependence. Of particular interest is physical dependence, which is characterized by a specific pattern of biological effects that occur when chronically administered opiates are withdrawn or displaced from their receptor complex. The need to relieve the physical distress of drug withdrawal has long been thought to be the most important motivational factor in drug abuse, since drug administration can abolish the withdrawal symptoms. However, a number of studies suggest that the development of physical dependence is not a condition sine qua non for opiates to be self-administered. Morphine will serve as a positive reinforcer at doses below those necessary to produce physical dependence determined by absence of withdrawal symptoms (51). A high degree of physical dependence induced by repeated administration of opiates hardly affects the acquisition of opiate self-administration (74). Brain mechanisms involved in opiate self-administration and in opiate-induced physical dependence are anatomically distinct from each other (7). Certain neuropeptides affect the development of opiate self-administration and that of physical dependence in an opposite direction (70). The self-administration of the endogenous opioid β-endorphin is accompanied by a very low level of physical dependence (75). Moreover, heroin can induce a conditioned place preference on the very first pairing of an environment with a heroin injection (7). These and other studies suggest that physical dependence is not a relevant variable for the reinforcing efficacy of opiates, although the withdrawal symptoms as a result of the presence of physical dependence may contribute to the maintenance or reevocation of opiate intake, and to its original level. Tolerance develops to a number of opiate effects upon repeated administration of these drugs. However, little or no tolerance appears to develop to the reinforcing effects and the discriminative internal stimuli of drugs (12,33). The acquisition of heroin self-administration is not significantly affected by manipulations aimed at inducing tolerance (74). Thus, tolerance may not be critically involved in the etiology of opiate self-administration. It seems that the positive reinforcing properties of opiates are the dominant determinants of the initiation and maintenance of their self-administration.

Internal Factors

Several techniques have been used to identify the neuronal substrate in the brain mediating the positive reinforcement of opiates. Self-administration of opiates is diminished by certain restricted brain lesions or by injecting opiate antagonists in dicrete brain regions (8,28). However, disrupting self-administration by these procedures does not mean that a brain structure in these regions is the site of opiate reward, because interference with any neuronal substrate along the pathways activated by the drug will affect self-administering behavior. The intracranial self-administration of opiates may be more promising in this respect. In experimentally naive rats, acquisition and maintenance of self-administration has been reported when opiates are microinjected into the ventral tegmental area (4,6,69). Such behavior is not observed when morphine is injected into the accumbal area, the lateral hypothalamic area, or the nucleus caudatus (4). Self-administration of opiates in some of these and other brain regions has been reported in another study, but the rats used were experienced in lever-pressing for brain stimulation reward (42). Opiate receptor antagonists injected into the ventral tegmental area or into the nucleus accumbens reduce intravenous heroin self-administration (8,59). Thus, neuronal elements present in the ventral tegmental area and the nucleus accumbens may be initial targets for opiates to produce reward. Conditioned place preference studies also indicate that these areas are important with respect to opiate reward (45,61). Opiates, like other drugs of abuse, affect rewarding brain stimulation. Although the initial reports suggested that opiates decreased the response rate of intracranial self-stimulation behavior (41), later studies demonstrated that opiates facilitate self-stimulation behavior, especially when response-rate-insensitive methods are used (23). Morphine dose dependently decreases the threshold for brain stimulation reward elicited from electrodes in the ventral tegmental area (77). Thus, the current evidence suggests that structures in the ventral tegmental area may be critically involved in the rewarding effects of opiates.

Central dopaminergic systems have been implicated in the mediation of reward, particularly the mesolimbic and mesocortical dopaminergic systems, with cell bodies in the ventral temental area and terminals in the nucleus accumbens and cortical areas, among others (25,81). It has indeed been shown that dopamine antagonists block place preference produced by heroin (5) and attenuate intravenous heroin self-administration (24). However, although heroin self-administration is diminished by systemic treatment with haloperidol, rather high doses of this drug are needed, which does not exclude aspecific effects (*unpublished data*). Moreover, microinjections of haloperidol in doses of 10 ng to 1 μg into the nucleus accumbens, the nucleus caudatus, the prefrontal cortex, the piriform cortex, or the amygdala do not interfere with intravenous heroin self-administration. Thus, when opiate reward is dependent on a dopaminergic system, the exact location of this system is yet unknown.

Other internal factors that may be involved in opiate reward and in the modulation of opiate self-administration are the pituitary hormones and neuropeptides, as will be discussed in the next section.

NEUROPEPTIDES AND OPIATE REWARD

The pituitary gland produces a number of peptide molecules, that is, hormones, that play an essential role in the homeostasis of the organism by controlling a variety of endocrine processes in the body, among others. During the past decades, evidence from behavioral, biochemical, and electrophysiological experiments was accumulating that these hormones are also implicated in brain processes (16,66). Interestingly, the peripheral endocrine action and the central action of these hormones can be dissociated. Thus, the classic endocrine effects need the whole or at least a major part of the molecule for full intrinsic activity, whereas the central effects can be mimicked by small parts, which are devoid of the endocrine activity of the parent hormone (15,16,66). These data indicate that the brain is a target organ for pituitary hormones. Peptide molecules affecting the nervous system are called neuropeptides. At present we know that pituitary hormones and a large number of other peptide molecules are formed throughout the CNS. They are likely present in peptidergic pathways. The neuropeptides generated in or outside these pathways by enzymes modulate neurotransmitter activity and, thereby, central brain functions. It has been postulated that disturbances in this control could result in psychopathology. The hormonal climate in the body and the brain neuropeptides may also be important for the initiation and maintenance of addiction to opiate and other drugs.

Vasopressin Neuropeptides

For our studies concerning the influence of neuropeptides on experimental addiction, we have selected intravenous heroin self-administration in rats. With this drug, self-injecting behavior develops relatively quickly and is rather reproducible, at least under standard conditions (68,74). We focused on acquisition of the behavior, since neuropeptides are involved in adaptation, and adaptive processes may play an important role in the mechanisms by which drug injection gains and maintains control over behavior. The peptide desglycinamide-[Arg8]vasopressin (DGAVP), which is much less potent than vasopressin with respect to antidiuretic and blood pressure increasing actions, decreases heroin intake during acquisition of intravenous self-administration when the peptide is administered subcutaneously, orally, or intracerebroventricularly (63,67,68). A similar effect has been found with [pGlu4,Cyt6]AVP-(4-8) (J. M. Van Ree, *unpublished data,* 1986), a recently discovered potent peptide, probably generated from vasopressin by brain enzymes (9). Vasopressin in the brain may play a physiological role in the behavior, since intracerebroventricularly injected antiserum against vasopressin, but not that against oxytocin or growth hormone, increased heroin self-administration (67). That rats refuse to exert more effort to obtain heroin when treated with DGAVP suggests that this peptide attenuates the reinforcing efficacy of the heroin injection (63). Evidence has been presented that the ventral tegmental area may be involved in the interaction between vasopressin neuropeptides and opiate reward. Thus, DGAVP decreases acquisition of fentanyl self-administration when this opiate is administered directly into the ventral tegmental area (69). Moreover, DGAVP attenuates intracranial electrical self-stimulation behavior elicited for that area (18). That this latter effect is present at threshold level of stimulation and not at high current intensity and that DGAVP does not decrease opiate intake during maintenance of heroin and morphine self-administration in rats and monkeys, respectively, (39,63) suggests that DGAVP is especially effective in situations in which the reinforcement control over self-injecting behavior is changed and/or the behavior is less strictly controlled. Such a situation may be present during the initial phase of the methadone detoxification program in mild to moderate heroin addicts. In two double-blind, placebo-controlled studies in which DGAVP was given during that initial phase a beneficial effect of peptide treatment has been found (26,60). Both heroin and cocaine use decrease by peptide treatment, which may suggest that the peptide has changed drug-seeking behavior in general.

Endorphins

Endorphins (endogenous morphine-like substances) mimic opiates in inducing a variety of behavioral effects ranging from immobility to behavioral activation. β-Endorphin is the most potent of these peptides when administered intracerebroventricularly in animals. The presence of endorphins in pituitary and brain has raised the question whether these entities are involved in the functioning of neuronal substrates affected by addictive drugs and mediate reinforcement. Thus, the endorphins may have intrinsic reinforcing efficacy and may mediate or modulate the reinforcing effect of opiates and other addictive drugs and of intracranial electrical selfstimulation. β-Endorphin supports self-administration when administered intracerebroventricularly (75). Also, the shorter endorphins, the enkephalins, and enkephalin analogs that are resistant to enzymatic activity have been shown to serve as reinforcers in naive and opiate-dependent animals (2,37,43,49,58). β-Endorphin and other opioid peptides possess discriminative internal stimulus properties similar to those of narcotic drugs (75,84). Conditioned place preference has been demonstrated with an enkephalin analog (46). Thus, endorphins and especially β-endorphin have intrinsic rewarding properties. Opiates may mimic these properties, and in this way, organisms may become dependent on the drugs. The involvement of endorphins in reward is supported by the attenuating influence of opiate antagonists on intracranial electrical self-stimulation (48). Opiate antagonists may especially be effective when the stimulus maintains rather low rates of lever-pressing and/or when the self-stimulation behavior is not yet fully developed (76), suggesting that endorphins modulate rather than mediate the reward from brain self-stimulation.

Other Neuropeptides

Some information is available that other pituitary hormones and related peptides interfere with opiate reward. Certain peptides related to ACTH-(4-10), especially γ_2-MSH, decrease acquisition of heroin self-injecting behavior in rats (64). This effect of γ_2-MSH may be related to the naloxone-like action of this peptide, as suggested from a number of other experiments (65). The C-terminal fragment of oxytocin (prolyl, leucyl, glycinamide) increased acquisition of heroin self-administration (68) and electrical brain self-stimulation elicited from the ventral tegmental area (18). Oxytocin and related peptides diminish heroin intake during maintenance of self-administration due probably to an attenuation of the tolerant state (36). Also, fragments of β-endorphin have been shown to affect opiate and brain reward. For example, the nonopioid and neurolepticum-like peptide des-Tyr¹-γ-endorphin decreases acquisition of heroin self-administration (64) and attenuates the electrical brain self-stimulation elicited from the ventral tegmental area and the nucleus accumbens (19,72). Prolactin lowers heroin intake during acquisition of drug self-administration (21), whereas intraventricularly injected antiserum to prolactin increases heroin intake (21,67). These data suggest that pituitary hormones and related neuropeptides are involved in and/or modulate brain processes implicated in acquisition and maintenance of opiate self-administration and of brain stimulation reward. In particular, mechanisms in the ventral tegmental area seem to be implicated in this respect. The various neuropeptides may thus play an important role in brain reward and opiate dependence and may contribute to the individual variation in susceptibility to opiate and other addictive drugs with respect to drug-taking behavior.

ENDORPHINS, REWARD, AND DEPENDENCE

The physiological role of the rewarding properties of endorphins, in particular β-endorphin, is not yet clear. One might speculate about euphoria, because the opiate-induced euphoria is thought to be a critical factor in the human abuse of opiates, which holds also for the rewarding properties of opiates. Euphoria is a feeling of well-being. Physiologically such a feeling is present during and/or after a delicious meal, enjoyable social contacts, a good performance, and sexual contacts, including orgasm, among others. There is indeed some evidence that endorphins play a role in these situations. Release of hypothalamic β-endorphin has been reported when rats eat highly palatable food (22). Endorphins may have a relation to the preference or aversiveness of food, and they may have a physiological regulatory role in the selection of food compounds (53). Manipulation of the opiate systems has marked effects on social interactions (44). Interestingly, low doses of β-endorphin increase social contacts of rats tested in dyadic encounters (71). The role of endorphins in sexual behavior may be more complex. In general, sexual activity may be decreased by opiates and β-endorphin (40). However, it has been suggested that endorphins may be released during sexual activity and may participate in orgasm, one positive reward from sexual fulfillment (31). Thus, endorphins, especially β-endorphin, may be implicated in these behaviors, which are accompanied by euphoria, and it may be postulated that this euphoria is at least partly mediated by the hedonistic action of these peptides.

However, the inherent reinforcing properties may also lead to development of dependence on behaviors probably associated with release of endorphins. This may be the underlying mechanism of certain addictive habits, like gambling and jogging. When a large amount of endorphins is released, euphoria may be changed to ecstasy, as is observed during or after some behaviors like ritualistic dancing ceremonies, which may induce a trance in which euphoria and analgesia are common symptoms (31). These data suggest that endorphins, particularly β-endorphin, may be a critical endogenous factor in addictive behavior in general. Accordingly, the endorphins have been implicated in dependence on drugs other than opiates. Blockade of opiate receptor systems with naltrexone decreases the reinforcing effects of ethanol in monkeys, the self-administering of ethanol via the intravenous route (1), and the amount of alcohol intake of rats subjected to a free-choice procedure to drink water and ethanol solutions (17). In alcoholics, the concentration of β-endorphin in the cerebrospinal fluid is markedly decreased as compared to that of normal individuals (27). Naloxone has been reported to reduce the amount of cigarettes smoked by chronic smokers (35), and smoking of nicotine is accompanied by secretion of β-endorphin into the bloodstream (47). Other endorphins, i.e., enkephalins, have been implicated in ethanol consumption of experimental animals (3). Thus, β-endorphin and the other endorphins may be common factors in addiction to various psychoactive drugs and habits. It should, however, be kept in mind that similar to the concept of multiple endogenous analgesic systems (79), multiple reward systems may be present in the brain in which endorphins may be implicated and in which endorphins are not primarily involved.

CONCLUDING REMARKS

The drug self-administration procedure in animals establishing the positive reinforcing properties of drugs has revealed that the rewarding action of drugs is a critical determinant of abuse liability and that this procedure can serve to predict qualitatively and quantitatively the abuse potential of drugs in humans. The procedure can be applied reliably to evaluate the variables that interfere with drug-taking behavior. Other procedures, such as the conditioned place preference and the interaction with brain stimulation reward, may also contribute to the understanding of the brain mechanisms underlying the rewarding action of drugs, including opiates.

Opiate reward can be elicited by drugs that have typical morphine-like actions. External factors, such as the dose of the drug, the schedule and conditions of drug availability, and stimulus control, are important for the initiation and maintenance of opiate self-administration. Although the development of tolerance and physical dependence may contribute more or less to opiate self-administrating behavior, these adaptive changes in the body are not critically involved in this behavior. Concerning the internal factors implicated in opiate reward, the available data suggest that mechanisms present in the ventral tegmental area are important in this respect. Whether these mechanisms include dopaminergic systems is not yet clear. Among the internal factors implicated in opiate reward are the pituitary hormones and neuropeptides. Under certain conditions, vasopressin and related peptides decrease heroin intake of experimental animals and humans and brain reward. The pituitary and brain endorphins, particularly β-endorphin, are candidates to play an essential role in reward processes and may be common factors in addiction to various psychoactive drugs and habits. Physiologically, endorphins, especially β-endorphin, may be implicated in euphoria, and, because of their inherent reinforcing properties, organisms may become dependent on behaviors associated with euphoria and the release of endorphins. Also other neuropeptides—e.g., those related to ACTH, including γ_2-MSH, and those related to prolactin and oxytocin—affect brain and opiate reward. Thus, disturbances in neuropeptide systems may lead to a state in which addictive behavior can easily be elicited and may be of relevance for the individual susceptibility to addictive drugs, including opiates. The demonstration of these disturbances in human addicts and their subsequent correction may yield a goal-directed treatment of addiction in the future.

REFERENCES

1. Altshuler, H. L., Phillips, P. E., and Feinhandler, D. A. (1980): Alteration of ethanol self-administration by naltrexone. *Life Sci., 26:*679–688.
2. Belluzzi, J. D., and Stein, L. (1977): Enkephalin may mediate euphoria and drive-reduction reward. *Nature,* 266:556–558.
3. Blum, K. (1984): Psychogenetics of drug seeking behavior. In: *Central and Peripheral Endorphins: Basic and Clinical Aspects,* edited by E. E. Müller and A. R. Genazzani, pp. 339–356. Raven Press, New York.
4. Bozarth, M. A. (1983): Opiate reward mechanisms mapped by intracranial self-administration. In: *The Neurobiology of Opiate Reward Processes,* edited by J. E. Smith and J. D. Lane, pp. 331–359. Elsevier Biomedical Press, Amsterdam.
5. Bozarth, M. A., and Wise, R. A. (1981): Heroin reward is dependent on a dopaminergic substrate. *Life Sci.,* 29:1881–1886.
6. Bozarth, M. A., and Wise, R. A. (1981): Intracranial self-administration of morphine into the ventral tegmental area in rats. *Life Sci.,* 28:551–555.
7. Bozarth, M. A., and Wise, R. A. (1983): Dissociation of the rewarding and physical dependence-producing properties of morphine. In: *Problems in Drug Dependence,* edited by L. S. Harris, pp. 171–177. NIDA, Rockville.
8. Britt, M. D., and Wise, R. A. (1983): Ventral tegmental site of opiate reward: Antagonism by a hydrophilic opiate receptor blocker. *Brain Res.,* 258:105–108.
9. Burbach, J. P. H., Kovács, G. L., De Wied, D., Van Nispen, J. W., and Greven, H. M. (1983): A major metabolite of arginine vasopressin in the brain is a highly potent neuropeptide. *Science,* 221:1310–1312.
10. Collins, R. J., Weeks, J. R., Cooper, M. M., Good, P. I., and Russell, R. R. (1984): Prediction of abuse liability of drugs using IV self-administration by rats. *Psychopharmacology (Berlin),* 82:6–13.
11. Colpaert, F. C. (1977): Narcotic cue and narcotic state. *Life Sci.,* 20:1097–1108.
12. Colpaert, F. C. (1978): Discriminative stimulus properties of narcotic analgesic drugs. *Pharmacol. Biochem. Behav.,* 9:863–887.
13. Colpaert, F. C., Niemegeers, C. J. E., and Janssen, P. A. J. (1976): The narcotic discriminative stimulus complex: Relation to analgesic activity. *J. Pharm. Pharmacol.,* 28:183–187.
14. Deneau, G., Yanagita, T., and Seevers, M. H. (1969): Self-administration of psychoactive substances by the monkey. *Psychopharmacologia,* 16:30–48.
15. De Wied, D. (1969): Effects of peptide hormones on behavior. In: *Frontiers in Neuroendocrinology,* edited by W. F. Ganong and L. Martini, pp. 97–140. Oxford University Press, New York.
16. De Wied, D., and Jolles, J. (1982): Neuropeptides derived from proopiocortin: Behavioral, physiological and neurochemical effects. *Physiol. Rev.,* 62:976–1059.
17. De Witte, P. (1984): Naloxone reduces alcohol intake in free-choice procedure even when both drinking bottles contain saccharin sodium or quinine substances. *Neuropsychobiology,* 12:73–77.
18. Dorsa, D. M., and Van Ree, J. M. (1979): Modulation of substantia nigra self-stimulation by neuropeptides related to neurohypophyseal hormones. *Brain Res.,* 172:367–371.
19. Dorsa, D. M., Van Ree, J. M., and De Wied, D. (1979): Effects of [Des-Tyr[1]]-γ-endorphin and α-endorphin on substantia nigra self-stimulation. *Pharmacol. Biochem. Behav.,* 10:899–905.
20. Downs, D. A., and Woods, J. H. (1976): Naloxone as a negative reinforcer in rhesus monkeys: Effects of dose, schedule, and narcotic regimen. *Pharmacol. Rev.,* 27:397–406.
21. Drago, F., and Scapagnini, U. (1985): Effects of endogenous hyperprolactinaemia on opiate-induced behavioral changes in rats. *Brain Res.,* 336:215–221.
22. Dum, J., Gramsch, C., and Herz, A. (1983): Activation of hypothalamic β-endorphin pools by reward induced by highly palatable food. *Pharmacol. Biochem. Behav.,* 18:443–447.
23. Esposito, R., and Kornetsky, C. (1977): Morphine lowering of self-stimulation thresholds: Lack of tolerance with long-term administration. *Science,* 195:189–191.

24. Ettenberg, A., Pettit, H. O., Bloom, F. E., and Koob, G. F. (1982): Heroin and cocaine intravenous self-administration in rats: Mediation by separate neural systems. *Psychopharmacology (Berlin),* 78:204–209.
25. Fibiger, H. C. (1978): Drugs and reinforcement mechanisms: A critical review of the catecholamine theory. *Annu. Rev. Pharmacol. Toxicol.,* 18:37–51.
26. Fraenkel, H. M., Van Beek-Verbeek, G., Fabriek, A. J., and Van Ree, J. M. (1983): Desglycinamide[9]-arginine[8]-vasopressin and ambulant methadone-detoxification of heroin addicts. *Alcohol Alcohol.,* 18:331–335.
27. Genazzani, A. R., Nappi, G., Facchinetti, F., Mazzella, G. L., Parrini, D., Sinforiani, E., Petraglia, F., and Savoldi, F. (1982): Central deficiency of β-endorphin in alcohol addicts. *J. Clin. Endocrinol. Metab.,* 55:583–586.
28. Glick, S. D., and Cox, R. D. (1977): Changes in morphine self-administration after brainstem lesions in rats. *Psychopharmacology (Berlin),* 52:151–156.
29. Grabowski, J., and Cherek, D. R. (1983): Conditioning factors in opiate dependence. In: *The Neurobiology of Opiate Reward Processes,* edited by J. E. Smith and J. D. Lane, pp. 175–210. Elsevier Biomedical Press, Amsterdam.
30. Headlee, C. P., Coppock, H. W., and Nichols, J. R. (1955): Apparatus and technique involved in a laboratory method of detecting the addictiveness of drugs. *J. Am. Pharm. Ass.,* 44:229–231.
31. Henry, J. L. (1982): Circulating opioids: Possible physiological roles in central nervous function. *Neurosci. Biobehav. Rev.,* 6:229–245.
32. Hofmeister, F. (1979): Progressive ratio performance in the rhesus monkey maintained by opiate infusions. *Psychopharmacology (Berlin),* 62:181–186.
33. Kalant, H. (1978): Behavioral criteria for tolerance and physical dependence. In: *The Bases of Addiction,* edited by J. Fishman, pp. 199–220. Dahlem Konferenzen, Berlin.
34. Kalant, H., Engel, J. A., Goldberg, L., Griffiths, R. R., Jaffe, J. H., Krasnegor, N. A., Mello, N. K., Mendelsohn, J. H., Thompson, T., and Van Ree, J. M. (1978): Behavioral aspects of addiction—Group report. In: *The Bases of Addiction,* edited by J. Fishman, pp. 463–496. Dahlem Konferenzen, Berlin.
35. Karras, A., and Kane, J. M. (1980): Naloxone reduces ciagerette smoking. *Life Sci.,* 27:1541–1545.
36. Kovács, G. L., and Van Ree, J. M. (1985): Behaviorally active oxytocin fragments simultaneously attenuate heroin self-administration and tolerance in rats. *Life Sci.,* 37:1895–1900.
37. Mello, N. K., and Mendelsohn, J. H. (1978): Self-administration of an enkephalin analog by rhesus monkey. *Pharmacol. Biochem. Behav.,* 9:579–586.
38. Mello, N. K., and Mendelsohn, J. H. (1978): Behavioral pharmacology of human alcohol, heroin and marihuana use. In: *The Bases of Addiction,* edited by J. Fishman, pp. 133–158. Dahlem Konferenzen, Berlin.
39. Mello, N. K., and Mendelson, J. H. (1979): Effects of the neuropeptide DG-AVP on morphine and food self-administration by dependent rhesus monkey. *Pharmacol. Biochem. Behav.,* 10:415–419.
40. Meyerson, B. I., and Terenius, L. (1977): β-Endorphin and male sexual behavior. *Eur. J. Pharmacol.,* 42:191–192.
41. Olds, J., and Travis, R. P. (1960): Effect of chlorpromazine, meprobamate, pentobarbital and morphine on self-stimulation. *J. Pharmacol. Exp. Ther.,* 128:397–404.
42. Olds, M. E. (1979): Hypothalamic substrate for the positive reinforcing properties of morphine in the rat. *Brain Res.,* 168:351–360.
43. Olds, M. E., and Williams, K. N. (1980): Self-administration of D-Ala[2]-met-enkephalinamide at hypothalamic self-stimulation sites. *Brain Res.,* 194:155–170.
44. Panksepp, J., Herman, B. H., Vilberg, T., Bishop, P., and DeEskinazi, F. G. (1980): Endogenous opioids and social behavior. *Neurosci. Biobehav. Rev.,* 4:473–487.
45. Philips, A. G., and LePaine, F. G. (1980): Reinforcing effects of morphine microinjections into the ventral tegmental area. *Pharmacol. Biochem. Behav.,* 12:965–968.
46. Philips, A. G., LePiane, F. G., and Fibiger, H. C. (1983): Dopaminergic mediation of reward produced by direct injection of enkephalin into the ventral tegmental area of the rat. *Life Sci.,* 33:2505–2511.
47. Pomerleau, O. F., and Pomerleau, C. S. (1984): Neuroregulators and the reinforcement of smoking: Towards a biobehavioral explanation. *Neurosci. Biobehav. Rev.,* 8:503–513.
48. Reid, L. D., and Siviy, S. M. (1983): Administration of opiate antagonists reveals endorphinergic

involvement in reinforcement processes. In: *The Neurobiology of Opiate Reward Processes,* edited by J. E. Smith and J. D. Lane, pp. 257–279. Elsevier Biomedical Press, Amsterdam.

49. Roemer, D., Buescher, H. H., Hill, R. C., Pless, J., Bauer, W., Cardinaux, F., Closse, A., Hauser, D., and Huguenin, R. (1977): A synthetic enkephalin analogue with prolonged parenteral and oral analgesic activity. *Nature,* 268:547–549.
50. Schuster, C. R., and Thompson, T. (1969): Self-administration of and behavioral dependence on drugs. *Annu. Rev. Pharmacol. Toxicol.,* 9:483–502.
51. Schuster, C. R., and Woods, J. H. (1968): The conditioned reinforcing effects of stimuli associated with morphine reinforcement. *Int. J. Addict.,* 3:223–230.
52. Shannon, H. E., and Holtzman, S. G. (1976): Evaluation of the discriminative effects of morphine in the rat. *J. Pharmacol. Exp. Ther.,* 198:54–65.
53. Siviy, S. M., and Reid, L. D. (1983): Endorphinergic modulation of acceptability of putative reinforcers. *Appetite J. Intake Res.,* 4:249–257.
54. Skinner, B. F. (1938): *The Behavior of Organisms.* Appleton-Century-Crofts, New York.
55. Spealman, R. D., and Goldberg, S. R. (1978): Drug self-administration by laboratory animals: Control by schedules of reinforcement. *Annu. Rev. Pharmacol. Toxicol.,* 18:313–339.
56. Spragg, S. D. S. (1940): *Comparative Psychology Monographs 15,* no. 7.
57. Thompson, T., and Unna, K. R. (1977): *Prediction of Abuse Liability of Stimulant and Depressant Drugs.* National Academy of Sciences–National Research Council, Washington.
58. Tortella, F. C., and Moreton, J. E. (1980): D-Ala^2-methionine-enkephalinamide self-administration in the morphine-dependent rat. *Psychopharmacology (Berlin),* 69:143–147.
59. Vaccarino, F. J., Bloom, F. E., and Koob, G. F. (1985): Blockade of nucleus accumbens opiate receptors attenuates intravenous heroin reward in the rat. *Psychopharmacology (Berlin),* 86:37–42.
60. Van Beek-Verbeek, G., Fraenkel, H. M., and Van Ree, J. M. (1983): Des-Gly^9-[Arg^8]-vasopressin may facilitate methadone detoxification of heroin addicts. *Subst. Alcohol Actions Misuse,* 4:375–382.
61. Van der Kooy, D., Mucha, R. F., O'Shaughnessy, M., and Bucenieks, P. (1982): Reinforcing effects of brain microinjections of morphine revealed by conditioned place preference. *Brain Res.,* 243:107–117.
62. Van Ree, J. M. (1979): Reinforcing stimulus properties of drugs. *Neuropharmacology,* 18:963–969.
63. Van Ree, J. M. (1982): Neurohypophyseal hormones and addiction. In: *Advances in Pharmacology and Therapeutics II, Vol. 1,* edited by H. Yoshida, Y. Hagihara, and S. Ebashi, pp. 199–209. Pergamon Press, Oxford.
64. Van Ree, J. M. (1983): The influence of neuropeptides related to proopiomelanocortin on acquisition of heroin self-administration of rats. *Life Sci.,* 33:2283–2289.
65. Van Ree, J. M., Bohus, B., Csontos, K. M., Gispen, W. H., Greven, H. M., Nijkamp, F. P., Opmeer, F. A., De Rotte, A. A., Van Wimersma Greidanus, T. B., Witter, A., and De Wied, D. (1981): Behavioral profiel of γ-MSH: Relationship with ACTH and β-endorphin action. *Life Sci.,* 28:2875–2888.
66. Van Ree, J. M., Bohus, B., Versteeg, D. H. G., and De Wied, D. (1978): Neurohypophyseal principles and memory processes. *Biochem. Pharmacol.,* 27:1793–1800.
67. Van Ree, J. M., and De Wied, D. (1977): Heroin self-administration is under control of vasopressin. *Life Sci.,* 21:315–320.
68. Van Ree, J. M., and De Wied, D. (1977): Modulation of heroin self-administration by neurohypophyseal principles. *Eur. J. Pharmacol.,* 43:199–202.
69. Van Ree, J. M., and De Wied, D. (1980): Involvement of neurohypophyseal peptides in drug-mediated adaptive responses. *Pharmacol. Biochem. Behav.,* 13(Suppl. 1):257–263.
70. Van Ree, J. M., and De Wied, D. (1981): Vasopressin, oxytocin and dependence on opiates. In: *Endogenous Peptides and Learning and Memory Processes,* edited by J. L. Martinez, R. A. Jensen, R. B. Messing, H. Rigter, and J. L. McGaugh, pp. 397–411. Academic Press, New York.
71. Van Ree, J. M., and Niesink, R. J. M. (1983): Low doses of β-endorphin increase social contacts of rats tested in dyadic encounters. *Life Sci.,* 33:611–614.
72. Van Ree, J. M., and Otte, A. P. (1980): Effects of (Des-Tyr^1)-γ-endorphin and α-endorphin as compared to haloperidol and amphetamine on nucleus accumbens self-stimulation. *Neuropharmacology,* 19:429–434.
73. Van Ree, J. M., Slangen, J. L., and De Wied, D. (1974): Self-administration of narcotic drugs

in rats: Dose-response studies. In: *Excerpta Medica Int. Congress Series No. 359,* pp. 231–239. Excerpta Medica, Amsterdam.
74. Van Ree, J. M., Slangen, J. L., and De Wied, D. (1978): Intravenous self-administration of drugs in rats. *J. Pharmacol. Exp. Ther.,* 204:547–557.
75. Van Ree, J. M., Smyth, D. G., and Colpaert, F. C. (1979): Dependence creating properties of lipotropin C-fragment (β-endorphin): Evidence for its internal control of behavior. *Life Sci.,* 24: 495–502.
76. Van Wolfswinkel, L., and Van Ree, J. M. (1985): Differential effect of naloxone on food and self-stimulation rewarded acquisition of a behavioral response pattern. *Pharmacol. Biochem. Behav.,* 23:199–202.
77. Van Wolfswinkel, L., and Van Ree, J. M. (1985): Effects of morphine and naloxone on thresholds of ventral tegmental electrical self-stimulation. *Naunyn Schmiedebergs Arch. Pharmacol.,* 330: 84–92.
78. Wallace, M., and Van Ree, J. M. (1981): Schedule induced self-injection of heroin: Dose response relationships. In: *Advances in Endogenous and Exogenous Opioids,* edited by H. Takagi and E. J. Simon, pp. 475–477. Elsevier Biomedical Press, Amsterdam.
79. Watkins, L. R., and Mayer, D. J. (1982): Organization of endogenous opiate and non-opiate pain control systems. *Science,* 216:1185–1192.
80. Weeks, J. (1962): Experimental morphine addiction: Method for automatic intravenous injection in unrestrained rats. *Science,* 138:143–144.
81. Wise, R. A. (1980): Action of drugs of abuse on brain reward systems. *Pharmacol. Biochem. Behav.,* 13(Suppl. 1):213–223.
82. Woods, J. H., Young, A. M., and Herling, S. (1982): Classification of narcotics on the basis of their reinforcing, discriminative, and antagonist effects in rhesus monkeys. *Fed. Proc.,* 41:221–227.
83. Young, A. M., Swain, H. H., and Woods, J. H. (1981): Comparison of opioid agonists in maintaining responding and in suppressing morphine withdrawal in rhesus monkeys. *Psychopharmacology (Berlin),* 74:329–335.
84. Young, A. M., Woods, J. H., Herling, S., and Hein, D. W. (1983): Comparison of the reinforcing and discriminative stimulus properties of opioids and opioid peptides. In: *The Neurobiology of Opiate Reward Processes,* edited by J. E. Smith and J. D. Lane, pp. 147–174. Elsevier Biomedical Press, Amsterdam.

Brain Reward Systems and Abuse, edited by
J. Engel and L. Oreland.
Raven Press, New York © 1987.

Mechanisms of PCP Action in the Central Nervous System

Michael R. Palmer, Yun Wang, Barry J. Hoffer,
and *Robert Freedman

*Departments of Pharmacology and *Psychiatry, University of Colorado Health Sciences
Center, Denver, Colorado 80262; and *Medical Research Service, Denver Veterans
Administration Medical Center, Denver, Colorado 80220*

Phencyclidine [1-(1-phenylcyclohexyl)-piperidine; PCP] and other arylcy-clohexylamines, such as ketamine and cyclohexylamine, were introduced as dissociative anesthetics (17,18,52). However, these agents have caused psychotic episodes in a significant proportion of patients (44). In addition, the positive reinforcing properties of PCP as well as the euphoria, amnesia, and other changes in mental state induced by this drug have, together with the general availability of PCP, led to its prominence as a major drug of abuse (12,26,29). By 1978, PCP abuse was recognized as a significant health problem in the United States (8). Although PCP congeners are often considered hallucinogens, their effects are not limited to the visual disturbances seen with LSD and mescaline. Instead, PCP use also can induce thought disorder, affective and behavioral changes, and disturbances of body image (6,15,23,30). The similarity of the symptoms of PCP-induced psychosis and acute schizophrenia has led to the classification of these agents as "schizophrenomimetic" or "psychotomimetic" (6,43,44), an analogy strengthened by the efficacy of antipsychotic drugs in ameliorating PCP-induced psychosis (44). The diversity and seriousness of the effects of PCP in humans have led to numerous investigations of its actions in the brain.

CHOLINERGIC MECHANISMS OF PCP ACTION

The anticholinergic action of PCP has been known for some time (1,20,46,58). Indeed, many of the central effects of PCP have been attributed to its anticholinergic action (38,45,46,73,75,76). PCP has been reported to reversibly block muscarinic cholinergic receptors (7,25,38,73). However, this is a relatively impotent action of PCP (73). Both electrophysiological and biochemical studies indicate that PCP blocks the nicotinic cholinergic ionophore at behaviorally relevent doses (4,21,37). This effect is apparently not due to a direct blockade of the receptor but rather to an allosteric interaction of PCP with loci on the receptor outside the acetyl choline (ACh) recognition site. The interactions of PCP with cholinergic synapses in the CNS, however, are not evenly distributed in all brain areas. In the hippocampus, for example, the electrophysiological effects of ACh are not directly altered by locally applied PCP (9). PCP alters ACh turnover in a number of brain regions, but the cholinergic systems in the hippocampus and in the striatum are not directly affected (55). Indeed, the PCP-induced inhibition of potassium-stimulated ACh release from striatal slices is apparently not due to a direct PCP interaction with the cholinergic synapse but rather to a PCP-induced release of dopamine (DA), which, in turn, inhibits ACh release in this preparation (40). A study of the rank order of potencies of various compounds for producing this effect indicate that it is not mediated through a PCP/sigma receptor, but, rather, this phenomenon might be mediated through a presynaptic δ opiate receptor (41). Thus, the PCP inhibition of ACh release can be blocked by both opiate and DA receptor antagonists. Interestingly, PCP increases ACh release in striatum in the presence of a DA blockade (41). This less prominent effect might be mediated through a PCP-induced blockade of potassium conductance, which has been reported to be associated with the direct actions of PCP at ACh receptors (2,3,5,39,72). This PCP-induced alteration of potassium channel function could effectively elongate the repolarization phase at the nerve terminal and, thus, could increase the amount of ACh released per nerve impulse.

ELECTROPHYSIOLOGICAL EVIDENCE FOR PRESYNAPTIC ACTIONS OF PCP ON CATECHOLAMINE NEUROTRANSMISSION

Because of the similarity between PCP-induced psychosis and schizophrenia, a brain dysfunction which is thought to involve aberrations in central noradrenergic and dopaminergic pathways (13,24), the interaction of PCP with catecholamines has been intensively investigated. The electrophysiological effects of locally applied PCP in the cerebellum are similar to the actions of norepinephrine (NE) in that brain area. Both PCP and ketamine cause depressions of the spontaneous firing rates when applied to single cerebellar Purkinje neurons by pressure ejection from multibarrel micropipettes (48,50). Similar to the relative behavioral potencies of these agents, PCP is 5- to 10-fold more potent than ketamine in this preparation. Similar to actions of NE in this brain area, the neuronal responses to PCP congeners are stereospecifically blocked by a number of antipsychotic drugs as well as by lithium applied either systemically or locally by pressure ejection. Although these data indicate that the cerebellar actions of PCP are mediated by a NE mechanism, PCP does not bind to catecholamine receptors (74,78). This might suggest that the locally applied PCP is activating noradrenergic synapses in the cerebellum. Supporting this hypothesis, PCP was found to be ineffective when neurotransmission is blocked (50,56). Furthermore, PCP is without effect on Purkinje neurons when the noradrenergic nerve terminals to cerebellum are lesioned with the catecholamine neurotoxin, 6-hydroxydopamine (6-OHDA). These data would suggest that a presynaptic interaction of PCP with

NE synapses appears to mediate PCP-induced depressions of cerebellar Purkinje neuron activity.

The actions of PCP in the hippocampus and in the caudate nucleus appear to be more complex. In both brain areas, locally applied PCP produced depressions of spontaneous activity of approximately 80% of the neurons encountered, although a small, but significant population of neurons is excited by this drug as well (10,31,64). In the hippocampus, the effects of PCP have been characterized on two different populations of neurons (64). While θ cells are encountered only infrequently, these neurons are excited by locally applied PCP. The firing rates of the more abundant complex-spike cells are depressed by PCP. Electrophysiological depressions of hippocampal pyramidal neurons by locally applied NE are mediated by α adrenergic mechanisms, whereas the NE-induced excitations are β mediated (54). Similarly, the PCP-induced depressions of the spontaneous activity of hippocampal pyramidal neurons can be reversibly blocked by locally applied phentolamine, an α adrenergic receptor antagonist, whereas the PCP-induced excitations were sensitive to the β adrenergic receptor blocker timolol (10). Thus, as was the case in the cerebellum, the electrophysiological actions of PCP in hippocampus appear to be mediated by noradrenergic mechanisms. Unlike in cerebellum, however, fluphenazine, an antipsychotic drug, did not alter the effects of PCP or NE in hippocampus (57). Consistent with the observation that PCP acts indirectly by elevating synaptically released levels of NE, the PCP-induced neuronal responses in hippocampus were reduced or eliminated after the depletion of the nerve terminal stores of catecholamines with reserpine (10) and after NE nerve terminals were selectively destroyed by the noradrenergic neurotoxin DSP4 (64).

Even though the neuronal responses to PCP in the caudate nucleus are more complex than in hippocampus or cerebellum, these effects are similar to those caused by local applications of DA in this brain area (31,32). PCP and DA have similar effects on caudate neuronal activity evoked by neocortical stimulation as well. The depressions but not the excitations of spontaneous neuronal activity in the caudate can be blocked by DA receptor antagonists (31,36). Thus, at least the PCP-induced depressions in this brain area appear to be mediated by a catecholamine mechanism. Furthermore, the effects of PCP but not DA were eliminated during the blockade of neurotransmission, as well as after neurotoxin lesions of the dopamine innervation of the caudate and after depletions of DA from caudate nerve terminals with reserpine. Thus, as was the case in the cerebellum and hippocampus, PCP-induced depressions of neuronal activity in the caudate appear to be indirectly mediated by catecholamine synapses as well.

MECHANISM OF THE PCP INTERACTION WITH CATECHOLAMINE SYNAPSES

The electrophysiological studies suggest that many of the actions of PCP in the CNS may be due to presynaptic effects of PCP on catecholamine nerve terminals (56), such as presynaptic induction of transmitter release, facilitation of ongoing transmitter release, or blockade of transmitter reuptake. PCP does not cause noradrenomimetic electrophysiological effects in the *in vitro* hippocampal slice (53). Because this preparation lacks intact spontaneously active NE afferents, this might suggest that PCP does not induce NE release in the hippocampus. However, PCP potentiates the electrophysiological effects of exogenously applied NE in this preparation (Dunwiddie, *unpublished data*, 1985). This is consistent with observations that PCP facilitates DA release from the caudate nucleus *in vitro* (33), similar to nonamphetamine stimulants (71). Micromolar doses of PCP specifically alter the calcium-independent release of the newly synthesized pool of DA without altering potassium-stimulated release of the catecholamine. The role, if any, of the reported PCP-induced blockade of DA reuptake in the striatum (27,70) in elevating calcium-independent release of DA is not currently understood. Increased synaptic levels of DA may activate feedback mechanisms that down-regulate DA synthesis in the nerve terminals *in vivo* (33). This latter mechanism might result in longer-term changes in DA transmitter system functions associated with chronic PCP use.

PCP INTERACTIONS WITH OTHER NEUROTRANSMITTER SYSTEMS

PCP and its congeners have been reported to interact with central adenosine mechanisms as well as to alter the function of a variety of neurotransmitter systems in the CNS (34). However, outside of the cholinergic and catecholaminergic interactions described above, there are few studies providing evidence for specific neurotransmitter mechanisms. Exceptions include the reported PCP-induced blockade of serotonin reuptake (68) and the interaction of PCP with various opiate receptors, in addition to the PCP/σ binding site, at higher drug concentrations (72,73,77,78). In addition, ketamine, a PCP analog, has been reported to selectively reduce polysynaptic reflexes in the spinal cord (14,69). This latter effect is probably mediated by a direct antagonism of postsynaptic actions of the excitatory amino acids released from these pathways. Iontophoretically applied ketamine causes a reversible and stereospecific antagonism of the electrophysiological excitations caused by local applications of L-aspartate (42). The responses to spinal reflex pathway were similarly affected. Excitations caused by kainate, quisqualate, and ACh, on the other hand, were either not affected by or were much less sensitive to ketamine.

ARE THE CNS EFFECTS OF PCP MEDIATED BY PCP/σ RECEPTORS?

A number of studies from different laboratories have indicated the presence of specific PCP binding sites in the brain (22,28,61,74,78). Evidence for the physiological significance of PCP binding is two-fold. First, there is a high correlation between the binding affinity of PCP congeners and benzomorphans *in vitro* and their biological activity *in vivo* (11,15,47,66,67). Second, an endogenous polypeptide ligand for the PCP receptor has been isolated (59,60). Thus, the PCP binding sites may well represent neurotransmitter receptors. There is evidence based on binding affinities and naloxone insensitivity that the σ "opiate" receptor is identical to the PCP binding site (28,61,79,80). Recently, however, evidence has been obtained for multiple binding sites for PCP-like compounds in the CNS (15,28,51,62,65). It is not clear at present, however, whether these sites represent a true diversity in PCP receptors or binding to a variety of opioid and cholinergic sites in addition to the σ receptor.

Although high doses of PCP and its congeners cause electrophysiological signs of local anesthesia (56,63), the stereoselectivity of behavioral (11,66,67) and elec-

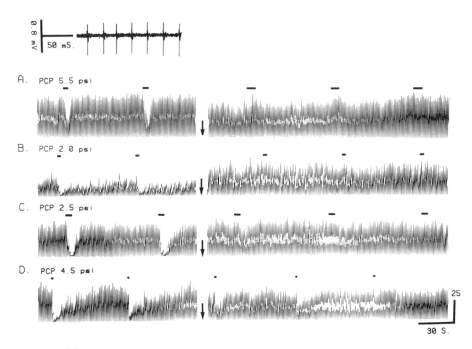

FIG. 1. Effects of local applications of metaphit on depressions from Purkinje neuron firing rate caused by pressure-ejected PCP. Firing rate is represented as action potentials/sec on the ordinate; time is represented on the abscissa in seconds. **A–D** represent four different cells. In each case, the PCP control responses are shown in the lefthand ratemeter record; the righthand records were acquired after metaphit application of 5 to 20 pounds/inch^2 (PSI) for 30 to 90 sec. Metaphit applications were continued until cell discharge was largely abolished; recovery of spontaneous activity then required 5 to 10 min, after which the PCP responses disappeared. This interval is indicated by the *break at the arrows*. Note that in **C** and **D**, the responses progressively diminish with time after metaphit. No recovery was observed as long as 30 to 60 min after metaphit application. **Inset** is an oscillographic record illustrating cerebellar action potential activity after recovery from a metaphit application.

trophysiological (10,35,42,49) responses to PCP/σ agonists suggests the receptor mediation of these effects. However, as was pointed out at the 1982 joint French–United States seminar on phencyclidine and related arylcyclohexylamines (19,34), the one missing criteria for PCP interactions to be considered receptor-mediated events was the demonstration of a specific antagonism of the pharmacological effects of PCP by a blocker of PCP binding sites. It was recently reported that an isothiocyanate derivative of PCP (metaphit) can produce a dose-dependent, irreversible antagonism of PCP binding to brain homogenates by acylating PCP binding sites (62). Metaphit has the same potency for inhibiting PCP-induced stereotypy and ataxia as for antagonizing PCP binding in the brain (16), although the ataxia obviously has a metaphit-insensitive component as well (15). The antagonism of the behavioral effects of PCP could be observed as long as 24 hr after metaphit treatment. We have recently found that locally applied metaphit irreversibly blocks PCP-induced depressions of the spontaneous firing rates of cerebellar Purkinje neurons (75) (Fig. 1). Similar depressions caused by locally applied NE and GABA were unaltered. Similarly, metaphit has been found to block irreversibly the electrophysiological effects of PCP, dexoxadrol, and (+)-cyclazocine in cerebellum (75; Y. Wang, M. Palmer, and R. Freedman, *unpublished data*), in hippocampus (Y. Wang, A. Pang, and B. Hoffer, *unpublished data*), and in the caudate nucleus (Johnson and Freedman, *unpublished data*). Both the binding data and the electrophysiological studies indicate that the PCP interactions in cerebellum are metaphit sensitive, whereas approximately 50% of the PCP actions in hippocampus and caudate are metaphit insensitive. Especially since it has been suggested that at least some of the PCP effects in the striatum are mediated by δ opioid receptors (41), it will be interesting to determine the nature of the metaphit-insensitive effects of PCP in these brain areas.

SUMMARY

The abuse potential and psychotomimetic properties of PCP and other dissociative anesthetics may be related to their interactions with DA neurotransmitter systems and reward pathways, as well as NE, serotonin, excitatory amino acids, and, perhaps, ACh. The effects of PCP are mediated through specific receptors. Although some of these effects involve PCP/σ binding sites, other receptor moieties may be involved as well. As is the case with adrenergic drugs, the receptor specificity of each behavioral or physiological effect may be dependent on the dose and receptor specificity of the pharmacological agent employed. Thus, whereas PCP might be more σ-specific at lower doses, other receptors may be activated as higher brain levels of the drug are reached. The intricacies of the potential interactions of various PCP effects in the CNS are further complicated by the observation that at least some PCP effects are dependent on the level of catecholaminergic synaptic activity. Thus, as one alters catecholamine transmitter release, the responses to PCP might also be changed. The multiple actions of

PCP detailed in this review are reflected in the numerous toxic effects, including psychosis, delirium and movement disorders, and abuse, which have been observed with both clinical and recreational use (6,30).

ACKNOWLEDGMENTS

The authors are supported by USPHS grants AA 05915 and DA 02429 and by a grant from the Veterans Administration Medical Research Service.

REFERENCES

1. Adams, P. M. (1980): Interaction of phencyclidine with drugs affecting cholinergic neurotransmission. *Neuropharmacology,* 19:151–153.
2. Aguayo, L. G., Warnick, J. E., Maayani, S., Glick, S. D., Weinstein, H., and Albuquerque, E. X. (1982): Sites of action of phencyclidine. IV. Interaction of phencyclidine and its analogues on ionic channels of the electrically excitable membrane and nicotinic receptor. Implications of behavioral effects. *Mol. Pharmacol.,* 21:637–647.
3. Albuquerque, E. X., Aguayo, L. G., Warnick, J. E., Weinstein, H., Glick, S. D., Maayani, S., Ickowicz, R. K., and Blaustein, M. P. (1981): The behavioral effect of phencyclidines may be due to their blockade of potassium channels. *Proc. Natl. Acad. Sci. USA,* 78:7792–7796.
4. Albuquerque, E. X., Tsai, M. C., Aronstam, R. S., Eldefrawi, A. T., and Eldefrawi, M. E. (1980): Sites of action of phencyclidine II. *Mol. Pharmacol.,* 18:167–178.
5. Albuquerque, E. X., Warnick, J. E., and Aguayo, L. G. (1983): Phencyclidine: Differentiation of behaviorally active from inactive analogs based on interactions with channels of electrically excitable membranes and of cholinergic receptors. In: *Phencyclidine and Related Arylcyclohexylamines: Present and Future Applications,* edited by J.-M. Kamenka, E. F. Domino, and P. Geneste, pp. 579–594. NPP Books, Ann Arbor.
6. Allen, R. M., and Young, S. J. (1978): Phencyclidine-induced psychosis. *Am. J. Psychiatry,* 135: 1081–1084.
7. Aronstam, R. S., Eldefrawi, M. E., Eldefrawi, A. T., Albuquerque, E. X., Jim, K. F., and Triggle, D. J. (1980): Site of action of phencyclidine III. *Mol. Pharmacol.,* 18:179–184.
8. Balster, R. L., and Pross, R. S. (1978): A bibliography of biomedical and behavioral research. *Journal of Psychedelic Drugs,* 10:1–15.
9. Bickford, P. C., Palmer, M. R., Hoffer, B. J., and Freedman, R. (1982): Interactions between phencyclidine and cholinergic excitation of hippocampal pyramidal neurons. *Neuropharmacology,* 21:729–732.
10. Bickford, P. C., Palmer, M. R., Rice, K. R., Hoffer, B. J., and Freedman, R. (1981): Electrophysiological effects of phencyclidine on rat hippocampal pyramidal neurons. *Neuropharmacology,* 20:733–742.
11. Brady, K. T., Balster, R. L., and May, E. L. (1982): Stereoisomers of *N*-allylnormetazocine: Phencyclidine-like behavioral effects in squirrel monkeys and rats. *Science,* 215:178–180.
12. Burns, R. S., and Lerner, S. E. (1976): Perspectives: Acute phencyclidine intoxication. *Clin. Toxicol.,* 9:477–501.
13. Carlsson, A. (1977): Dopaminergic autoreceptors: Background and implications. In: *Advances in Biochemical Psychopharmacology, Vol. 16,* edited by E. Costa and G. L. Gessa, pp. 439–441. Raven Press, New York.
14. Chen, G., and Chow, S. Y. (1975): Effects of ketamine on synaptic transmission in cat spinal cord. *Neuropharmacology,* 14:147–149.
15. Contreras, P. C., and O'Donohue, T. L. (1985): Stereotyped behavior correlates better than ataxia with phencyclidine-receptor interactions. *Eur. J. Pharmacol. (in press).*
16. Contreras, P. C., Rafferty, M. C., Jacobson, A. E., Rice, K. C., Quirion, R., and O'Donohue, T. L. (1984): Agonist and antagonist effects of PCP derivatives on binding and behavior. *Society for Neuroscience Abstracts,* 10:1205.
17. Corssen, G., Miyasaka, M., and Domino, E. F. (1968): Changing concepts in pain control during surgery: Dissociative anesthesia with CI-581, a progress report. *Anesth. Analg.,* 47:745–759.

18. Domino, E. F. (1964): Neurobiology of phencyclidine (Sernyl), a drug with an unusual spectrum of pharmacological activity. *Int. Rev. Neurobiol.,* 6:303–347.
19. Domino, E. F., Kamenka, J.-M., and Geneste, P. (1983): The joint French-US seminar on phencyclidine and related arylcyclohexylamines. *Trends in Pharmacolog. Sci.,* 9:363–367.
20. Domino, E. F., and Wilson, A. E. (1972): Psychotropic drug influences on brain acetylcholine utilization. *Psychopharmacology (Berlin),* 25:291–298.
21. Eldefrawi, M. E., Eldefrawi, A. T., Aronstam, R. S., Warnick, S. E., and Albuquerque, E. X. (1980): [^{3}H]Phencyclidine: A probe for the ionic channel of the nicotinic receptor. *Proc. Natl. Acad. Sci. USA,* 77:7458–7462.
22. Eldefrawi, A. T., Miller, E. R., Murphy, D. R., and Eldefrawi, M. E. (1982): (^{3}H)-Phencyclidine interactions with the nicotinic acetylcholine receptor channel and its inhibition by psychotropic, opiate, antidepressant, antibiotic, antiviral, and antiarrhythmic drugs. *Mol. Pharmacol.,* 22:72–81.
23. Fessler, R. B., Sturgeon, R. D., and Meltzer, H. Y. (1979): Phencyclidine-induced ipsilateral rotation in rats with unilateral 6-hydroxydopamine-induced lesions of the substantia nigra. *Life Sci.,* 24:1281–1288.
24. Freedman, R. (1977): Interactions of antipsychotic drugs with norepinephrine and cerebellar neuronal circuitry: Implications for the physiology of psychosis. *Biol. Psychiatry,* 12:181–196.
25. Gabrielevitz, A., Kloog, Y., Kalir, A., Balderman, D., and Sokolovsky, M. (1980): Interaction of phencyclidine and its new adamantyl derivatives with muscarinic receptors. *Life Sci.,* 26:89–95.
26. Gallant, D. M., and Mallott, D. B. (1983): Overview of the human behavioral psychopharmacology of the cyclohexylamines. In: *Phencyclidine and Related Arylcyclohexylamines: Present and Future Applications,* edited by J.-M. Kamenka, E. F. Domino, and P. Geneste, pp. 563–571. NPP Books, Ann Arbor.
27. Gerhardt, G., and Rose, G. (1985): Presynaptic action of phencyclidine (PCP) in the rat striatum defined using *in vivo* electrochemical methods. *Society for Neuroscience Abstracts,* 11:2105.
28. Hampton, R. Y., Medzihradsky, F., Woods, J. H., and Dahlstrom, P. J. (1982): Stereospecific binding of ^{3}H-phencyclidine in rat brain membranes. *Life Sci.,* 30:2147–2154.
29. Ingold, F. R. (1983): PCP and substance dependency. In: *Phencyclidine and Related Arylcyclohexylamines: Present and Future Applications,* edited by J.-M. Kamenka, E. F. Domino, and P. Geneste, pp. 573–578. NPP Books, Ann Arbor.
30. Jaffe, J. H. (1985): Drug addiction and drug abuse. In: *Goodman and Gilman's The Pharmacological Basis of Therapeutics,* edited by A. G. Gilman, L. S. Goodman, T. W. Rall, and F. Murad, pp. 532–581. MacMillan Publishing Company, New York.
31. Johnson, S. W., Haroldsen, P. E., Hoffer, B. J., and Freedman, R. (1984): Presynaptic dopaminergic activity of phencyclidine in rat caudate. *J. Pharmacol. Exp. Ther.,* 229:322–332.
32. Johnson, S. W., Palmer, M. P., and Freedman, R. (1983): Effects of dopamine on spontaneous and evoked activity of caudate neurons. *Neuropharmacology,* 22:843–851.
33. Johnson, K. M., Vicroy, T. W., Leventer, S. M., and Mok, L. S. (1983): Phencyclidine: Effects on striatal dopaminergic and cholinergic systems. In: *Phencyclidine and Related Arylcyclohexylamines: Present and Future Applications,* edited by J.-M. Kamenka, E. F. Domino, and P. Geneste, pp. 83–106. NPP Books, Ann Arbor.
34. Kamenka, J.-M., Domino, E. F., and Geneste, P. (1983): *Phencyclidine and Related Arylcyclohexylamines: Present and Future Applications.* NPP Books, Ann Arbor.
35. Kim, M., Pang, K., Freedman, R., and Palmer, M. (1985): Electrophysiological effects of cyclazocine on rat cerebellar Purkinje neurons: Comparison with phencyclidine. *Alcohol Drug Res.,* 6:23–26.
36. Kirch, D. G., Palmer, M. R., Egan, M., and Freedman, R. (1985): Electrophysiological interactions between haloperidol and reduced haloperidol, and dopamine, norepinephrine and phencyclidine in rat brain. *Neuropharmacology,* 24:375–379.
37. Kloog, Y., Gabrielevitz, A., Kalir, A., Balderman, D., and Sokolovsky, M. (1979): Functional evidence for a second binding site of nicotinic antagonists using phencyclidine derivatives. *Biochem. Pharmacol.,* 28:1447–1450.
38. Kloog, Y., Rehavi, M., Maayani, S., and Sokolovsky, M. (1977): Anticholinesterase and antiacetylcholine activity of 1-phenylcyclohexylamine derivatives. *Eur. J. Pharmacol.,* 45:221–227.
39. Lazdunski, M., Bidard, J.-N., Romey, G., Tourneur, Y., Vignon, J., and Vincent, J.-P. (1983): The different sites of action of phencyclidine and its analogues in nervous tissues. In: *Phencyclidine and Related Arylcyclohexylamines: Present and Future Applications,* edited by J.-M. Kamenka, E. F. Domino, and P. Geneste, pp. 83–106. NPP Books, Ann Arbor.

40. Leventer, S. M., and Johnson, K. M. (1983): Effects of phencyclidine on the release of radioactivity from rat striatal slices labeled with [³H]choline. *J. Pharmacol. Exp. Ther.,* 225:332–336.
41. Leventer, S. M., and Johnson, K. M. (1984): Phencyclidine-induced inhibition of striatal acetylcholine release: Comparisons with mu, kappa, and sigma opiate agonists. *Life Sci.,* 34:793–801.
42. Lodge, D., Anis, N. A., Berry, S. C., and Burton, N. R. (1983): Arylcyclohexylamines selectively reduce excitation of mammalian neurones by aspartate-like amino acids. In: *Phencyclidine and Related Arylcyclohexylamines: Present and Future Applications,* edited by J.-M. Kamenka, E. F. Domino, and P. Geneste, pp. 595–616. NPP Books, Ann Arbor.
43. Luby, E. D., Cohen, B. D., Rosenbaum, G., Gottleib, J. S., and Kelley, R. (1959): Study of a new schizophrenomimetic drug, Sernyl. *Arch. Neurol. Psychiatry,* 31:363–369.
44. Luisada, P. B., and Brown, B. I. (1976): Clinical management of the phencyclidine psychosis. *Clin. Toxicol.,* 9:539–543.
45. Maayani, S., and Weinstein, H. (1979): Some structure activity relationships of phencyclidine derivatives as anticholinergic agents *in vitro* and *in vivo.* In: *Membrane Mechanisms of Drugs of Abuse,* edited by C. Sharp and L. G. Abood, pp. 91–106. Alan R. Liss, New York.
46. Maayani, S., Weinstein, A., Ben-Zvi, N., Cohen, S., and Sokolovsky, M. (1974): Psychotomimetics as anticholinergic agents. I. 1-Cyclohexylpiperidine derivatives: Anticholinesterase activity and antagonistic activity to acetylcholine. *Biochem. Pharmacol.,* 23:1263–1281.
47. Martin, W. R., Eades, C. G., Thompson, J. A., Huppler, R. E., and Gilbert, P. E. (1976): The effects of morphine- and nalorphine-like drugs in the nondependent and morphine-dependent chronic spinal dog. *J. Pharmacol. Exp. Ther.,* 197:517–532.
48. Marwaha, J., Palmer, M., Hoffer, B., and Freedman, R. (1980): Phencyclidine-induced depressions of cerebellar Purkinje neurons. *Life Sci.,* 26:1509–1515.
49. Marwaha, J., Palmer, M., Hoffer, B., Freedman, R., Rice, K. C., Paul, S., and Skolnick, P. (1981): Differential electrophysiological and behavioral responses to optically active derivatives of phencyclidine. *Arch. Pharmacol.,* 315:203–209.
50. Marwaha, J., Palmer, M. P., Woodward, D. J., Hoffer, B. J., and Freedman, R. (1980): Electrophysiological evidence for presynaptic actions of phencyclidine on noradrenergic terminals in rat cerebellum. *J. Pharmacol. Exp. Ther.,* 215:606–613.
51. Mendelshon, L. G., Derchner, G. A., Kalra, V., Zimmerman, D. M., and Leander, J. D. (1984): Phencyclidine receptors in rat brain cortex. *Biochem. Pharmacol.,* 33:3529–3535.
52. Miyasaka, M., and Domino, E. F. (1968): Neuronal mechanisms of ketamine-induced anesthesia. *Int. J. Neuropharmacol.,* 7:557–573.
53. Mueller, A. L., Kirk, K. L., Hoffer, B. J., and Dunwiddie, T. V. (1982): Noradrenergic responses in rat hippocampus: Electrophysiological actions of direct- and indirect-acting sympathomimetics in the *in vitro* slice. *J. Pharmacol. Exp. Ther.,* 223:599–605.
54. Mueller, A. L., Palmer, M. R., Hoffer, B. J., and Dunwiddie, T. V. (1982): Hippocampal noradrenergic responses in vivo and in vitro: Characterization of alpha and beta components. *Naunyn Schmiedebergs Arch. Pharmacol.,* 318:259–266.
55. Murray, T. F. (1983): A comparison of phencyclidine with other psychoactive drugs on cholinergic dynamics in the rat brain. In: *Phencyclidine and Related Arylcyclohexylamines: Present and Future Applications,* edited by J.-M. Kamenka, E. F. Domino, and P. Geneste, pp. 547–561. NPP Books, Ann Arbor.
56. Palmer, M. R., Bickford, P. C., Hoffer, B. J., and Freedman, R. (1983): Electrophysiological evidence for presynaptic actions of phencyclidine on noradrenergic transmission in rat cerebellum and hippocampus. In: *Phencyclidine and Related Arylcyclohexylamines: Present and Future Applications,* edited by J.-M. Kamenka, E. F. Domino, and P. Geneste, pp. 443–469. NPP Books, Ann Arbor.
57. Palmer, M. R., Freedman, R., and Dunwiddie, T. V. (1982): Interactions of a neuroleptic drug (fluphenazine) with catecholamines in hippocampus. *Psychopharmacology (Berlin),* 76:122–129.
58. Petersen, R. C., and Stillman, R. C. (1978): Phencyclidine: An overview. In: *Phencyclidine (PCP) Abuse: An Appraisal. National Institute of Drug Abuse Research Monograph 21,* edited by R. C. Petersen and R. C. Stillman, pp. 1–27. National Institute of Drug Abuse, Rockville, Maryland.
59. Quirion, R., DiMaggio, D. A., French, E. D., Contreras, P. C., Shiloach, J., Pert, C. B., Everist, H., Pert, A., and O'Donohue, T. L. (1984): Evidence for an endogenous peptide ligand for the phencyclidine receptor. *Peptides (Fayetteville),* 5:967–974.
60. Quirion, R., O'Donohue, T. L., Everist, H., Pert, A., and Pert, C. B. (1983): Phencyclidine receptors and possible existence of an endogenous ligand. In: *Phencyclidine and Related Aryl-*

cyclohexylamines: Present and Future Applications, edited by J.-M. Kamenka, E. F. Domino, and P. Geneste, pp. 667–684. NPP Books, Ann Arbor.
61. Quirion, R., Rice, K. C., Skolnick, P., Paul, S., and Pert, C. B. (1981): Stereospecific displacement of (^{3}H)-phencyclidine (PCP) receptor binding by an enantiomeric pair of PCP analogs. *Eur. J. Pharmacol.,* 74:107–108.
62. Rafferty, M. F., Mattson, M., Jacobson, A. E., and Rice, K. C. (1985): A specific acylating agent for the [^{3}H]phencyclidine receptors in rat brain. *Fed. Eur. Biochem. Soc. Lett.,* 181:318–322.
63. Raja, S. N., and Gueyenet, P. G. (1980): Effects of phencyclidine on the spontaneous activity of monoaminergic neurons. *Eur. J. Pharmacol.,* 62:229–233.
64. Rose, G., Pang, K., Palmer, M., and Freedman, R. (1984): Differential effects of phencyclidine upon hippocampal complex-spike and theta neurons. *Neurosci. Lett.,* 45:141–146.
65. Sethy, V. H., and McCall, J. M. (1984): High-affinity (^{3}H)-dexoxadrol binding to rat brain membranes. *Drug. Develop. Res.,* 4:635–645.
66. Shannon, H. E. (1983): Discriminative stimulus effects of phencyclidine: Structure-activity relationships. In: *Phencyclidine and Related Arylcyclohexylamines: Present and Future Applications,* edited by J.-M. Kamenka, E. F. Domino, and P. Geneste, pp. 311–335. NPP Books, Ann Arbor.
67. Slifer, B. L., and Balster, R. L. (1983): Reinforcing properties of stereoisomers of the putative *sigma* agonists N-allylnormetazocine and cyclazocine in Rhesus monkeys. *J. Pharmacol. Exp. Ther.,* 225:522–528.
68. Smith, R. C., Meltzer, H. Y., Arora, R. C., and Davis, J. M. (1977): Effects of phencyclidine on [^{3}H]catecholamine and [^{3}H]serotonin uptake in synaptosomal preparations from rat brain. *Biochem. Pharmacol.,* 26:1435–1439.
69. Tang, A. H., and Schroeder, L. A. (1973): Spinal cord depressant effects of ketamine and dexoxadrol in the cat and the rat. *Anesthesiology,* 39:37–43.
70. Vickroy, T. W., and Johnson, K. M. (1980): *In vivo* administration of phencyclidine inhibits ^{3}H-dopamine accumulation by rat brain striatal slices. *Subst. Alcohol Actions Misuse,* 1:351–354.
71. Vickroy, T. W., and Johnson, K. M. (1982): Similar dopamine-releasing effects of phencyclidine and non-amphetamine stimulants in striatal slices. *J. Pharmacol. Exp. Ther.,* 223:669–674.
72. Vincent, J.-P., Bidard, J.-N., Lazdunski, M., Romey, G., Tourneur, Y., and Vignon, J. (1983): Identification and properties of phencyclidine-binding sites in nervous tissues. *Fed. Proc.,* 42:2570–2573.
73. Vincent, J.-P., Cavey, D., Kamenka, J.-M., Geneste, P., and Lazdunski, M. (1978): Interaction of phencyclidine with the muscarinic and opiate receptors in the central nervous system. *Brain Res.,* 152:176–182.
74. Vincent, J.-P., Kartalovski, B., Geneste, P., Kamenka, J.-M., and Lazdunski, M. (1979): Interaction of phencyclidine ("angel dust") with a specific receptor in rat brain membranes. *Proc. Natl. Acad. Sci. USA,* 79:4678–4682.
75. Wang, Y., Palmer, M., Freedman, R., Hoffer, B., Mattson, M., Lessor, R. A., Rafferty, M. F., Rice, K. C., and Jacobson, A. E. (1986): Electrophysiological and biochemical study of the antagonism of PCP action by metaphit in rat cerebellar Purkinje cells. *Proc. Natl. Acad. Sci. USA,* 83:2724–2727.
76. Weinstein, H., Maayani, S., Glick, S. D., and Meibach, R. C. (1981): Integrated studies on the biochemical, behavioral, and molecular pharmacology of phencyclidine: A progress report. In: *PCP (Phencyclidine): Historical and Current Perspectives,* edited by E. F. Domino, pp. 131–175. NPP Books, Ann Arbor.
77. Zukin, S. R. (1982): Differing stereospecificities distinguish opiate receptor subtypes. *Life Sci.,* 31:1307–1310.
78. Zukin, S. R., and Zukin, R. S. (1979): Specific [^{3}H] phencyclidine binding in rat central nervous system. *Proc. Natl. Acad. Sci. USA,* 76:5372–5376.
79. Zukin, R. S., and Zukin, S. R. (1981): Multiple opiate receptors: Emerging concepts. *Life Sci.,* 29:2681–2690.
80. Zukin, R. S., and Zukin, S. R. (1983): A common receptor for phencyclidine and the *sigma* opiates. In: *Phencyclidine and Related Arylcyclohexylamines: Present and Future Applications,* edited by J.-M. Kamenka, E. F. Domino, and P. Geneste, pp. 107–124. NPP Books, Ann Arbor.

Brain Reward Systems and Abuse, edited by
J. Engel and L. Oreland.
Raven Press, New York © 1987.

Interactions of Ethanol with Opiate Receptors: Implications for the Mechanism of Action of Ethanol

Boris Tabakoff and Paula L. Hoffman

*National Institute on Alcohol Abuse and Alcoholism, Laboratory for Studies of
Neuroadaptive Processes, National Institutes of Health, Bethesda, Maryland 20205*

It is assumed that ethanol is ingested for its pharmacologic effects and that certain of these effects are reinforcing and will tend to maintain ethanol consumption (1). However, although self-administration of ethanol can be demonstrated in animals (1,54), there are quantitative and qualitative differences between the reinforcing properties of ethanol and other drugs that are abused. The major differences can be explained by ethanol's lack of potency as a reinforcer: that is, ethanol must be ingested or administered at much higher doses than other abused drugs in order to observe reinforcing or other effects. At these high doses, the aversive (tissue-irritating) effects of ethanol or its metabolite acetaldehyde may counter the positive reinforcing effects (52). Thus, the balance between an individual's sensitivity to the positively reinforcing effects of ethanol and to its aversive effects may be important for determining the initial overall level of reinforcement produced by ethanol in that individual (52).

One reason that high doses of ethanol may be required to produce reinforcement, as well as other physiological effects, is that ethanol, unlike most other drugs of abuse, does not interact with specific receptors in the CNS. It has been known for some time, however, that ethanol can partition into and disrupt the structure of neuronal cell membranes (5,14,45). The membrane "fluidizing" effects of ethanol have also been shown to correlate positively with the sensitivity of animals to the hypnotic effect of ethanol (11). Therefore, it has been postulated that the neuronal cell membrane represents the initial site of action of ethanol in the CNS. On the other hand, while lipids represent the structural moieties of neuronal membranes, membrane-bound proteins, such as receptors, enzymes, and ionophores, are the functional components of the membranes, and these proteins essentially control synaptic transmission. The activity of the membrane-bound proteins is influenced by the properties of the lipids that immediately surround them (e.g., refs. 10 and 30), and, thus, ethanol could affect the activities of the proteins directly or secondarily by its effects on membrane lipid properties.

The lipid microdomain of each protein may vary in lipid composition and sensitivity to ethanol, and this variation could lend specificity to the effects of ethanol, leading to selective biochemical and behavioral responses.

One receptor system that has been implicated in the reinforcing effects of ethanol is the opiate receptor. For example, the opiate receptor antagonist naltrexone was reported to reduce ethanol self-administration by monkeys, suggesting that opiate receptors may mediate the rewarding effects of ethanol (1). Similarly, it was reported that naloxone, another opiate receptor antagonist, blocked the facilitatory effect of ethanol on responding for hypothalamic self-stimulation by rats (33). Opiate receptor antagonists have also been reported to reverse ethanol-induced coma (13,23,26,35) or prevent symptoms of ethanol intoxication (22,47). However, these latter findings are more controversial (15,32,37), and it is not clear if all of the effects of naloxone are related to its action at opiate receptors (44).

Nevertheless, interest in the possible interactions of ethanol and opiate systems has led to several studies of the effects of ethanol on opiate receptor binding. The results of these studies not only indicate that ethanol can selectively affect the properties of various opiate receptor subtypes in brain but also contribute to a more general model for understanding the effects of ethanol on membrane-bound receptor systems.

The acute, *in vitro* effects of ethanol on opiate receptor binding have been studied in several laboratories. Hiller et al. (16) reported that ethanol selectively inhibited the binding of ^{3}H-[2-D-Ala,5-D-Leu]enkephalin (ENK) to δ opiate receptors (i.e., receptors with high affinity for ENK) in membranes derived from whole rat brain. These investigators also observed a slight stimulation of ^{3}H-dihydromorphine (DHM) binding to μ receptors (receptors with high affinity for morphine) in the same tissue. This stimulation was evident at relatively high (>200 mM) concentrations of ethanol. In these studies, ethanol did not affect the binding of naloxone or ethylketocyclazocine (a ligand that is relatively selective for κ receptors). More recently, Hiller et al. (17) found that 1-butanol had effects similar to ethanol, in that ligand binding to κ receptors was not affected, and enkephalin binding to δ receptors was inhibited. Gianoulakis also found that ethanol stimulated DHM binding, inhibited ENK binding, and had no effect on naloxone binding (12). Since naloxone may bind essentially equally to μ and δ receptors, it was suggested that the lack of effect of ethanol on antagonist binding resulted from the balance of stimulatory and inhibitory effects on ligand binding to μ and δ receptors (12). Jørgenson and Hole (24) also found that ethanol had no effect on the binding of etorphine, an agonist that does not distinguish between μ and δ receptors, to rat brain membranes. The major difference between the studies of Hiller et al. (16,17) and those of Gianoulakis (12) was that the former attributed the effects of ethanol on opiate binding to changes in receptor affinity, whereas the latter found changes in receptor number.

In striatal tissue from mice, ethanol was also shown to differentially affect ligand binding to μ and δ receptors (50). When assays were carried out at 25°C, ethanol had a biphasic effect on DHM binding to striatal tissue. A low concentration of ethanol (50 mM) stimulated binding, whereas higher concentrations inhibited binding. All concentrations of ethanol inhibited ENK binding, and, as had been reported for rat brain, ethanol was a more potent inhibitor of ligand binding to the δ receptor, as opposed to the μ receptor. It was demonstrated that ethanol inhibited striatal opiate binding in a pseudocompetitive manner; i.e., ethanol appeared to change the affinity of the receptor for ligand. Thus, the ligand concentration used for assessing the effects of ethanol is important, since, when only a single ligand concentration is used, the effectiveness of ethanol to inhibit binding depends on this concentration (50). The use of high ligand concentrations (higher than the K_D concentration) may account in part for the reports by Hiller et al. (16) and Jørgenson and Hole (24) that ethanol did not inhibit DHM or etorphine binding. On the other hand, ligand binding to κ receptors appears to be insensitive to ethanol, regardless of ligand concentration used (17; S. Khatami, P. L. Hoffman, B. Tabakoff, and B. P. Salafsky, *unpublished observation,* 1985), and the higher sensitivity of δ receptors than of μ receptors was not solely a result of the ligand concentration used (50).

Other factors that influence the effect of *in vitro* ethanol on opiate receptor binding include the assay temperature and the presence of ions or guanine nucleotides in the assay mixtures. At 37°C, in mouse striatal tissue, the affinity of μ and δ receptors for DHM and ENK, respectively, was decreased, as compared to 25°C, and ethanol no longer stimulated DHM binding (18). Ethanol was more potent at inhibiting the binding of both ligands at 37°C than at 25°C, presumably as a result of the decreased affinity of the receptors for their ligands at 37°C, since the same concentration of each ligand was used at both temperatures (18).

Sodium ion (Na^+) and guanosine triphosphate (GTP) are believed to promote the coupling of opiate receptors to adenylate cyclase (2,9,27,28; and see below) and, in so doing, to alter the binding of ligands to opiate receptors (4,38). GTP affects binding via an interaction with the guanine nucleotide binding protein, N_i (25,49), while the effect of Na^+ on ligand binding may result from a direct action at the receptor, e.g., a change in receptor conformation (8). GTP reduces the affinity of opiate receptors for ligands (4,38), while Na^+ has been reported to reduce both affinity and number of binding sites (21,29,46). The effects of ethanol and other alcohols on opiate receptor binding are altered in the presence of GTP or Na^+. These compounds potentiate the effects of the alcohols on ligand binding to μ and δ receptors in mouse striatal (18) and rat brain membranes (17). The presence of ions, if not taken into account, may also contribute to differences between studies. For example, Levine et al. (31), in contrast to others (12,16,24), reported that ethanol increased the number of binding sites for naloxone in membranes from whole rat brain. The binding studies of Levine et al. (31), however, were carried out in the presence of 100 mM NaCl, which was not included in the other studies.

In general, it appears that ethanol *in vitro* inhibits opiate receptor binding by decreasing the affinity of the receptors for ligands; this action is enhanced at physiological temperature and in the presence of endogenous "coupling factors."

The effect of ethanol may be mediated by its ability to perturb or fluidize neuronal membrane lipids, since the potency of short-chain alcohols to inhibit binding was linearly related to their carbon chain length (16,17). Similarly, it has been demonstrated that the potency of alcohols to perturb lipid properties is linearly related to the chain length (36). However, even if mediated by lipid perturbation, the effects of ethanol are selective. The δ opiate receptor seems to be more sensitive to ethanol than other opiate receptor subtypes. This sensitivity could result from the specific lipid composition of the membrane microdomain of the δ receptor or from the characteristics of the receptor protein itself.

The finding that both GTP and ethanol decreased opiate receptor affinity for ligands (4,38,50) and that the effect of ethanol on opiate receptor binding was potentiated by GTP (18) suggested that ethanol and GTP might alter opiate binding by similar mechanisms. Opiate agonists inhibit the activity of adenylate cyclase (AC) (2,9,19,20,27,28), and as mentioned earlier, GTP is required in order to couple opiate receptors to AC. The opiate receptor–AC system appears to consist of at least three proteins: the receptor, the inhibitory nucleotide binding protein, N_i (25), and the catalytic unit of the enzyme. The interactions among these proteins lead to the inhibition of AC activity. The model describing these interactions is based on that developed for systems in which neurotransmitters or hormones *stimulate* AC, but, for the most part, the mechanisms for stimulation and inhibition seem similar (48,49). According to this model, the neurotransmitter interacts with a low-affinity form of the receptor, which then interacts with N_s (the stimulatory nucleotide binding protein) or N_i, forming a ternary complex in which the receptor has high affinity for the ligand (48,49). The guanine nucleotide binding proteins, N_s and N_i, consist of three subunits (α, β, and γ) (7). The β/γ subunits of N_i and N_s are identical, while the α subunits differ. GTP binds to α_s or α_i, inducing dissociation of the ternary complex and reversion of the receptor to its low-affinity state. Thus, in ligand binding studies, one can discern high- and low-affinity binding sites for agonists in the absence of GTP; in its presence, only low-affinity binding is detectable (48,49). The effect of GTP on opiate binding seems to conform to this model, for the most part, since GTP appears to lower the affinity of opiate receptors for ligands.

The interactions of N_i and N_s with AC to produce activation or inhibition of enzyme activity may be somewhat different (7). The α_s subunit of N_s with GTP bound interacts with the catalytic unit of AC to induce activation (48,49). There is some evidence that α_i may interact in a similar manner to cause inhibition (7). However, there is also evidence to suggest that the β/γ subunit of N_i might interact with the α_s subunit of N_s to produce inhibition of AC (7).

It has been demonstrated that ethanol stimulates AC activity in striatum as well as cerebral cortex of mice (34,40,41,43). In striatum, ethanol was proposed to alter the equilibrium between α_s and AC to favor formation of the activated complex (34). In cortex, ethanol had a similar action but also acted at other sites: ethanol affected the β-adrenergic receptor and promoted the dissociation of N_s (43). Ethanol also had a slight activating effect on the catalytic unit of cerebral cortical AC (43). The sites of action of ethanol in these systems are specific, but the effect of ethanol appears to depend, in part, on changes in membrane lipid properties (34). Because ethanol affected opiate binding in a similar manner to GTP and because of the effects of ethanol in the stimulatory AC systems, it seemed likely that ethanol, perhaps by altering membrane fluidity and thus the interactions of membrane-bound proteins, would also affect opiate inhibition of AC.

In striatum, the δ opiate receptor is coupled to AC. This was demonstrated by assessing the relative potencies of various opiates to inhibit enzyme activity (9,28) and by the finding that the peptide morphiceptin, which binds selectively to μ opiate receptors, did not inhibit AC activity (19). However, although ethanol inhibited ENK binding to striatal δ receptors and, in fact, this receptor subtype was the most sensitive to the effects of ethanol (16,50), ethanol had no effect on the inhibition of mouse striatal AC by enkephalin or by morphine (20). There are several possible explanations for these results. One is suggested by the work of Childers and LaRiviere (3), who found that the effects of GTP on opiate receptor binding and on the coupling of receptors to AC may be mediated by different guanine nucleotide binding proteins. If this is the case, ethanol could independently affect opiate binding and inhibition of AC activity by specific effects on different proteins. Another possible explanation is that the receptors that are detected in ligand binding studies are different from the receptors that are coupled to AC.

The finding that ethanol did not alter opiate inhibition of AC was also surprising because of the data, discussed above, showing that ethanol does modulate the activity of striatal systems in which neurotransmitters stimulate AC (34,40,41). Since the actions of ethanol in these systems were suggested to be mediated by effects on membrane lipid fluidity (34), the finding that ethanol did not affect inhibition of striatal AC by opiates could be interpreted to support the hypothesis that changes in membrane fluidity do not affect movement of all protein components within the membrane in the same way. As discussed earlier, it is possible that different proteins (e.g., N_s and N_i) may exist in differing lipid microdomains within the membrane, which are more or less sensitive to ethanol. An alternative explanation is that ethanol specifically modulates the activity of N_s as opposed to N_i. This possibility is supported by preliminary studies indicating that ethanol also does not modify inhibition of striatal AC by cholinergic agonists (B. Tabakoff, C. T. Chung, and P. L. Hoffman, *unpublished observations, 1986*).

In any case, it seems clear that, although ethanol does alter opiate binding to striatal receptors, it would not interfere with any physiological effects of opiates that are mediated by coupling of the δ receptors to AC. However, opiates have other biochemical effects that do not appear to involve AC activity. For example, opiates are known to modulate Ca^{2+} mobilization and neurotransmitter release (6). In mouse striatum, it has been demonstrated that opiates can stimulate the synthesis and release of the neurotransmitter dopamine (DA) (53,56), although it is not clear which opiate receptor subtype is associated with this action. Dopaminergic systems have been implicated in the mechanism of ethanol-induced reinforcement (52,55), and modulation of opiate effects on DA could contribute to this reinforcement. Although *striatal* DA systems may not be crucial for the reinforcing properties of ethanol and other drugs (52,55), this system provides a useful model for assessing opiate/DA interactions and the effects of ethanol on these interactions. Studies of the acute interactions of ethanol and opiates on DA release can be difficult to interpret, since ethanol itself may alter DA release or, particularly in *in vivo* studies, may interact with several neuronal systems that modulate DA release (51). However, investigations of the effect of chronic ethanol administration on opiate receptors and on the effects of opiates on DA release have provided evidence that ethanol can alter opiate receptor–effector coupling processes.

Since ethanol acutely altered opiate binding and selectively affected certain opiate receptor subtypes, it was of interest to determine whether chronic ingestion or administration of ethanol would also affect opiate receptor binding and whether subtypes of opiate receptors would respond differentially to this treatment. It is clear that under physiological conditions (i.e., at 37°C, in the presence of guanine nucleotide or Na^+), concentrations of ethanol that can be attained *in vivo* had significant effects on opiate receptor binding (18). Therefore, after chronic ethanol ingestion, one might expect to see cumulative changes in receptor properties or adaptive responses of the receptors to the initial effect of ethanol, especially in animals that develop tolerance and/or physical dependence on ethanol. When rats were fed a liquid diet containing ethanol for 3 weeks, increased affinity of the δ receptor for ENK, decreased affinity of the μ receptor for DHM, and an increase in B_{max} for all ligands (ENK, DHM, and naloxone) in brain membranes were reported (12). In this study, a decreased effect of ethanol added *in vitro* on opiate binding to tissues of ethanol-fed animals, as compared to those of controls, was also observed, suggesting the development of tolerance at the biochemical level (12). In rats given ethanol in their drinking water for 3 weeks, the affinity for ENK of the δ receptor in membranes of the forebrain was increased, and no change in μ receptor properties was observed (39). The increase in δ receptor affinity could represent an adaptation to the initial acute effect of ethanol, which was to lower the affinity of the δ receptor for ENK. In this study (39), assays were performed in the presence of 100 mM NaCl, whereas in the former study with rats (12), NaCl was not used, which may account for some of the discrepancies. The importance of NaCl, particularly for evaluating μ receptor properties, was illustrated in a study done with mice (21). Mice were fed a liquid diet containing ethanol for 7 days, at which time they were tolerant to and physically dependent on ethanol (42). Striatal opiate receptor binding was assessed at 24 hr after withdrawal from ethanol ingestion, when ethanol had been eliminated and overt withdrawal signs had dissipated. It was found that the affinity of the striatal μ receptor for DHM was reduced (21), whereas there was no change in the properties of the striatal δ receptor for ENK (S. Urwyler and B. Tabakoff, *unpublished observations*, 1981). These assays were performed in the absence of

Na$^+$. When Na$^+$ was included in the assays, it was found that the μ receptor in the ethanol-withdrawn mice, which already showed low affinity for DHM, was also less sensitive to the effect of Na$^+$ on affinity than the μ receptor in control mice (21). That is, if Na$^+$ is a coupling factor for opiate receptors, the μ receptor in the ethanol-withdrawn mice may have been in an uncoupled state, insensitive to Na$^+$. If all assays had been performed in the presence of Na$^+$ no change in the properties of the μ receptor would have been apparent, similar to what was reported in rat brain in the presence of Na$^+$ (39). Although Na$^+$ is generally believed to play a role in the coupling of inhibitory receptors to AC, as mentioned above, μ receptors are not coupled to AC. Furthermore, opiate inhibition of AC was not altered in animals chronically treated with ethanol (20), as might have been expected, since ethanol did not affect this system acutely (20). However, when the effect of morphine on striatal DA synthesis and release was determined in ethanol-withdrawn mice, the dose–response curve for this effect was shifted to the right, as compared to that in controls (21), consistent with the decreased affinity for morphine of the striatal μ receptor. This result is also consistent with the hypothesis that the μ receptor may be uncoupled from its effector (21) in ethanol-withdrawn mice. These findings support the hypothesis that, in the mouse, μ opiate receptors are coupled to DA synthesis and release, and ethanol can selectively modulate the activity of this receptor–effector coupling system. Decreased function of striatal μ opiate receptors or receptors which modulate DA release in other brain areas following chronic ethanol ingestion could well play a role in the development of tolerance to the reinforcing effect of ethanol.

The studies of the effects of ethanol on opiate receptor function illustrate the specificity and selectivity of the actions of ethanol in the brain. These findings, in conjunction with results on the effects of ethanol on other neurotransmitter receptor–effector coupling systems (7,34,40,41,43), allow a better understanding of the specific sites and mechanisms of action of ethanol in the CNS, which lead to specific physiological effects, including intoxication, tolerance and physical dependence, and perhaps reinforcement.

REFERENCES

1. Altshuler, H. L. (1976): Intragastric self-administration of ethanol: A subhuman primate model of alcoholism. In: *Animal Models in Alcohol Research,* edited by K. Ericksson, J. P. Sinclair, and K. Kiianma, pp. 179–184. Academic Press, New York.
2. Blume, A. J., Lichshtein, D., and Boone, G. (1979): Coupling of opiate receptors to adenylate cyclase: Requirement for Na$^+$ and GTP. *Proc. Natl. Acad. Sci. USA,* 76:5626–5630.
3. Childers, S. R., and LaRiviere, G. (1984): Modification of guanine nucleotide-regulatory components in brain membranes. *J. Neurosci.,* 4:2764–2771.
4. Childers, S. R., and Snyder, S. H. (1980): Differential regulation by guanyl nucleotides of opiate agonist and antagonist receptor interactions. *J. Neurochem.,* 34:583–593.
5. Chin, J. H., and Goldstein, D. B. (1977): Effects of low concentrations of ethanol on the fluidity of spin-labeled erythrocyte and brain membranes. *Mol. Pharmacol.,* 13:435–441.
6. Clouet, D. H. (1977): Neurochemical aspects of opiate dependence: An overview. In: *Alcohol and Opiates. Neurochemical and Behavioral Mechanisms,* edited by K. Blum, pp. 237–254. Academic Press, New York.

7. Codina, J., Hildebrandt, J., Sunyer, T., Sekura, R. D., Manclark, C. R., Iyengar, R., and Birn-baumer, L. (1984): Mechanisms in the vectorial receptor-adenylate cyclase signal transduction. *Adv. Cyclic Nucleotide Protein Phosphorylation Res.,* 17:111–125.
8. Cooper, D. M. F. (1982): Bimodal regulation of adenylate cyclase. *FEBS Lett.,* 138:157–163.
9. Cooper, D. M. F., Londos, C., Gill, D. L., and Rodbell, M. (1982): Opiate receptor-mediated inhibition of adenylate cyclase in rat striatal plasma membranes. *J. Neurochem.,* 38:1164–1167.
10. Farias, R. N., Bloj, B., Morero, R. D., Siñeriz, F., and Trucco, R. E. (1975): Regulation of allosteric membrane-bound enzymes through changes in membrane lipid composition. *Biochim. Biophys. Acta,* 415:231–251.
11. Goldstein, D. B., Chin, J. H., and Lyon, R. C. (1982): Ethanol-disordering of spin-labeled mouse brain membranes: Correlation with genetically-determined ethanol sensitivity of mice. *Proc. Natl. Acad. Sci. USA.,* 79:4231–4233.
12. Gianoulakis, C. (1983): Long-term ethanol alters the binding of ^{3}H-opiates to brain membranes. *Life Sci.,* 33:725–733.
13. Guerin, J. M., and Friedberg, G. (1982): Naloxone and ethanol intoxication. *Ann. Intern. Med.,* 97:932.
14. Harris, R. A., and Schroeder, F. (1981): Ethanol and the physical properties of brain membranes: Fluorescence studies. *Mol. Pharmacol.,* 20:128–137.
15. Hemmingsen, R., and Sorenson, S. C. (1980): Absence of an effect of naloxone on ethanol intoxication and withdrawal reaction. *Acta Pharmacol. Toxicol. (Copenh.),* 46:62–65.
16. Hiller, J. M., Angel, L. M., and Simon, E. J. (1981): Multiple opiate receptors: Alcohol selectively inhibits binding to delta receptors. *Science,* 214:468–469.
17. Hiller, J. M., Angel, L. M., and Simon, E. J. (1984): Characterization of the selective inhibition of the *delta* subclass of opioid binding sites by alcohols. *Mol. Pharmacol.,* 25:249–255.
18. Hoffman, P. L., Chung, C. T., and Tabakoff, B. (1984): Effects of ethanol, temperature and endogenous regulatory factors on the characteristics of striatal opiate receptors. *J. Neurochem.,* 43:1003–1010.
19. Hoffman, P. L., Luthin, G. R., Theodoropoulos, D., Cordopatis, P., and Tabakoff, B. (1983): Ethanol effects on striatal dopamine receptor-coupled adenylate cyclase and on striatal opiate receptors. *Pharmacol. Biochem. Behav.,* 18(Suppl. 1):355–359.
20. Hoffman, P. L., and Tabakoff, B. (1986): Ethanol does not modify opiate-mediated inhibition of striatal adenylate cyclase. *J. Neurochem., 46:812–816.*
21. Hoffman, P. L., Urwyler, S., and Tabakoff, B. (1982): Alterations in opiate receptor function after chronic ethanol treatment. *J. Pharmacol. Exp. Ther.,* 222:182–189.
22. Jeffcoate, W. J., Herbert, M., Cullen, M. H., Hastings, A. G., and Walder, C. P. (1979): Prevention of the effects of alcohol intoxication by naloxone. *Lancet,* 2:1157–1159.
23. Jefferys, D. B., Flanagan, R. F., and Volans, G. N. (1980): Reversal of ethanol-induced coma by naloxone. *Lancet,* 1:308–309.
24. Jørgensen, H., and Hole, K. (1981): Does ethanol stimulate brain opiate receptors? Studies on receptor binding and naloxone inhibition of ethanol-induced effects. *Eur. J. Pharmacol.,* 75: 223–229.
25. Katada, T., Bokoch, G. M., Northup, J. K., Michio, U., and Gilman, A. G. (1984): The inhibitory guanine nucleotide-binding regulatory component of adenylate cyclase. Properties and function of the purified protein. *J. Biol. Chem.,* 259:3568–3577.
26. Khanna, J. M., Mayer, J. M., Kalant, H., and Shah, G. (1982): Effect of naloxone on ethanol- and pentobarbital-induced narcosis. *Can. J. Physiol. Pharmacol.,* 60:1315–1318.
27. Law, P. Y., Koehler, J. E., and Loh, H. H. (1982): Comparison of opiate inhibition of adenylate cyclase activity in neuroblastoma N18TG2 and neuroblastoma × glioma NG108-15 hybrid cell lines. *Mol. Pharmacol.,* 21:483–491.
28. Law, P. Y., Wu, J., Koehler, J. E., and Loh, H. H. (1981): Demonstration and characterization of opiate inhibition of the striatal adenylate cyclase. *J. Neurochem.,* 36:1834–1846.
29. Lee, C.-Y., Akera, T., and Brody, T. M. (1977): Effects of Na$^+$, K$^+$, Mg^{++} and Ca^{++} on the saturable binding of [^{3}H]dihydromorphine and [^{3}H]naloxone *in vitro. J. Pharmacol. Exp. Ther.,* 202:166–173.
30. Lenaz, G., Curatola, G., and Masotti, L. (1975): Perturbation of membrane fluidity. *J. Bioenerg. Biomembr.,* 7:223–299.
31. Levine, A. S., Hess, S., and Morley, J. E. (1983): Alcohol and the opiate receptor. *Alcoholism: Clin. Exp. Res.,* 7:83–84.

32. Lignian, H., Fontaine, J., and Askenasi, R. (1983): Naloxone and alcohol intoxication in the dog. *Hum. Toxicol.,* 2:221–225.
33. Lorens, S. A., and Sainati, S. M. (1978): Naloxone blocks the excitatory effect of ethanol and chlordiazepoxide on lateral hypothalamic self-stimulation behavior. *Life Sci.,* 23:1359–1364.
34. Luthin, G. R., and Tabakoff, B. (1984): Activation of adenylate cyclase by alcohols requires the nucleotide-binding protein. *J. Pharmacol. Exp. Ther.,* 228:579–587.
35. Lyon, L. J., and Antony, J. (1982): Reversal of alcohol coma by naloxone. *Ann. Intern. Med.,* 96:464–465.
36. Lyon, R. C., McComb, J. A., Schreurs, J., and Goldstein, D. B. (1984): A relationship between alcohol intoxication and the disordering of brain membranes by a series of short-chain alcohols. *J. Pharmacol. Exp. Ther.,* 218:669–675.
37. Mattila, M. J., Nuomo, E., and Sepalla, T. (1981): Naloxone is not an effective antagonist of ethanol. *Lancet,* 1:775–776.
38. Pfeiffer, A., Sadee, W., and Herz, A. (1980): Differential regulation of the μ, δ and κ-opiate receptor subtypes by guanyl nucleotides and metal ions. *J. Neurosci.,* 2:912–917.
39. Pfeiffer, A., Seizinger, B. R., and Herz, A. (1981): Chronic ethanol inhibition interferes with δ, but not with μ, opiate receptors. *Neuropharmacology,* 20:1229–1232.
40. Rabin, R. A., and Molinoff, P. B. (1981): Activation of adenylate cyclase by ethanol in mouse striatal tissue. *J. Pharmacol. Exp. Ther.,* 216:129–134.
41. Rabin, R. A., and Molinoff, P. B. (1983): Multiple sites of action of ethanol on adenylate cyclase. *J. Pharmacol. Exp. Ther.,* 227:551–556.
42. Ritzmann, R. F., and Tabakoff, B. (1976): Body temperature in mice: A quantitative measure of alcohol tolerance and physical dependence. *J. Pharmacol. Exp. Ther.,* 199:158–170.
43. Saito, T., Lee, J. M., and Tabakoff, B. (1985): Ethanol's effects on cortical adenylate cyclase activity. *J. Neurochem.,* 44:1037–1044.
44. Sawynok, J., Pinsky, C., and LaBella, F. S. (1979): Minireview on the specificity of naloxone as an opiate antagonist. *Life Sci.,* 25:1621–1632.
45. Seeman, P. (1972): The membrane actions of anesthetics and tranquilizers. *Pharmacol. Rev.,* 24:583–655.
46. Simon, E. J., Hiller, J. M., Groth, J., and Edelman, I. (1975): Further properties of stereospecific opiate binding sites in rat brain: On the nature of the sodium effect. *J. Pharmacol. Exp. Ther.,* 192:531–537.
47. Sorenson, S. C., and Mattison, K. (1978): Naloxone as an antagonist in severe alcohol intoxication. *Lancet,* 2:688–689.
48. Spiegel, A. M., Gierschik, M. D., Levine, M. A., and Downs, R. W., Jr. (1985): Clinical implications of guanine nucleotide-binding proteins as receptor-effector couplers. *N. Engl. J. Med.,* 312:26–33.
49. Stadel, J. M., deLean, A., and Lefkowitz, R. J. (1982): Molecular mechanisms of coupling in hormone receptor–adenylate cyclase systems. *Adv. Enzymol.,* 53:1–43.
50. Tabakoff, B., and Hoffman, P. L. (1983): Alcohol interactions with brain opiate receptors. *Life Sci.,* 32:192–204.
51. Tabakoff, B., and Hoffman, P. L. (1983): Neurochemical aspects of tolerance to and physical dependence on alcohol. In: *The Biology of Alcoholism, Vol. 7,* edited by B. Kissin and H. Begleiter, pp. 199–252. Plenum Press, New York.
52. Tabakoff, B., and Hoffman, P. L.: A neurobiological theory of alcoholism. In: *Theories of Alcoholism,* edited by C. D. Chaudron and D. A. Wilkinson. Addiction Research Foundation, Toronto (*in press*).
53. Urwyler, S., and Tabakoff, B. (1981): Stimulation of dopamine synthesis and release by morphine and D-Ala-2-D-Leu-5-enkephalin in the mouse striatum *in vivo. Life Sci.,* 28:2277–2286.
54. Winger, G. D., and Woods, J. H. (1973): The reinforcing property of ethanol in the Rhesus monkey: I. Initiation, maintenance and termination of intravenous ethanol-reinforced responding. *Ann. N.Y. Acad. Sci.,* 215:162–175.
55. Wise, R. A. (1980): Actions of drugs of abuse on brain reward systems. *Pharmacol. Biochem. Behav.,* 18(Suppl. 1):213–223.
56. Wood, P. L., Stotland, M., Richard, J. W., and Rackham, A. (1980): Actions of mu, sigma, delta and agonist/antagonist opiates on striatal dopaminergic function. *J. Pharmacol. Exp. Ther.,* 215:697–703.

Brain Reward Systems and Abuse, edited by
J. Engel and L. Oreland.
Raven Press, New York © 1987.

Clinical Effects of Central Nervous System Stimulants: A Selective Update

Burton Angrist

*Department of Psychiatry, New York University Medical Center and Veterans
Administration Medical Center, New York, New York 10010*

This chapter will both summarize and attempt to update information covered in past reviews (2,7). Factors that might modify clinical responses to CNS stimulants such as genetic variables, dose, route of administration, tolerance, and supersensitivity will be considered first, followed by discussion of the clinical effects of the drugs themselves.

VARIABILITY OF RESPONSE TO CNS STIMULANTS

The variability of individual responses to CNS stimulants has been a source of perplexity throughout the history of these agents. In 1884, Freud likened the effects of cocaine in himself to a physiological sense of well-being. Just 3 years later, when adverse effects occurred in others after similar doses to those he had taken, he questioned whether the "reason for the irregularity of the cocaine effect lies in individual variations in excitability" (21).

Similarly, shortly after amphetamine was introduced, Reifenstein and Davidoff (46) described seizures and unconsciousness after doses as low as 30 mg, although other patients had taken 150 mg daily for 6 months without untoward effects.

In a more recent review, Kalant (30) described a woman who developed a sense of impending death, frontal headaches, palpitations, and retrosternal discomfort after only 5 mg *d*-amphetamine by mouth and another who, after receiving 10 mg amphetamine intravenously, "began to scream that she was being watched and that the doctor wanted to kill her on orders from the Church." Conversely, in the same review, another woman was described who took 630 mg *d*-amphetamine orally when depressed and became only "mildly excited but easily calmed by reassurance." Higher individual doses have, of course, been frequently reported by CNS stimulant abusers.

Although these are rather extreme examples, this wide variation in dose and effect is certainly striking and perhaps greater than is seen with any other class of drugs.

FACTORS AFFECTING THE CLINICAL RESPONSE TO CNS STIMULANTS

Possible Genetic Determinants of CNS Stimulant Response

Differences in the behavior of several strains of mice were observed in the 1940s and 1950s (38). Neurochemical studies of these strains were first reported in 1962. These initially focused on serotonin levels rather than on the catecholaminergic systems considered to mediate response to CNS stimulants (38). However, thereafter, genetic differences in regional brain norepinephrine content were described (52,61). Genetic differences in catecholamine systems were more strongly suggested in 1972 when Ciaranello et al. (14) demonstrated strain-dependent differences in tyrosine hydroxylase activity. Genetic variation in the response to amphetamine has now specifically been shown by both Garrattini et al. (22) and Reis et al. (47). Garrattini et al. (22) showed that animals with higher dopamine turnover were more sentitive to a variety of behavioral and neurochemical effects of amphetamine. Reis et al. (47) showed that differences in brain organization and number of dopaminergic neurons constituted a basis for variance in sensitivity to the effects of amphetamine on locomotion and in inducing stereotypy.

Clinical studies in this area were lacking until 1981, when Nurnberger et al. (40) evaluated the effects of amphetamine in 13 identical twin pairs. Responses differed widely between the pairs but were strikingly concordant within each pair and were generally not correlated with plasma amphetamine levels. These findings suggested that the pharmacodynamic responsivity to CNS stimulants is to some degree under genetic control in humans.

Dosage

In individuals whose response to stimulants is not idiosyncratically unusual, dosage is the most critical determinant of stimulant effects. Characteristic feelings of a minimal effective dose of CNS stimulants include feelings of "relaxed" alertness, energetic vitality, and confident assertiveness. Appetite and fatigue disappear, and the person is not inclined to eat and cannot sleep. These effects would be noted by most people, for example, at doses of 2.5 to 15 mg of *d*-amphetamine.

With somewhat larger doses (e.g., 20 to 50 mg amphetamine), all effects are intensified, but the initial sense of "relaxed" alertness is replaced by a "driven" feeling. Dysphoric feelings become admixed with euphoria. Thoughts become rapid. Emotions become more labile and intense, and a sense of earnestness and decreased frivolity are often felt. Impulsivity increases, and, as in hypomania, priorities are often not ordered appropriately. These effects combined with increased talkativeness, intrusiveness, and a predilection for somewhat inappropriately personal topics of conversation frequently make individuals who have taken such doses tiresome to others.

Very high doses of CNS stimulants are incompatible with normal social functioning and also carry the liabilities of severely disturbed behavior, psychosis, and a severe degree of dependence. Some individuals take moderately high doses of stimulants on a more or less daily basis and suffer these consequences to varying degrees. Alternatively, a pattern of cyclic use emerges when the drug is taken in binges separated by periods of recovery. Such users experience cycles of unproductive, frenzied activity, stereotypy, or psychosis alternating with exhaustion, extended sleep, and a period of dysphoric lethargy thereafter (33). It is interesting to note that both rats and monkeys given free access to amphetamine and other CNS stimulants in intravenous self-adminstration experiments tend to evolve a similar cyclic pattern of use (41,54).

Route of Administration

The immediate subjective effects of intravenously administered CNS stimulants (or inhalation of cocaine base) are intense and dramatic. Rylander had provided a vivid description of the effects of intravenous phenmetrazine (51) as follows: "One of the addicts . . . said that at first he feels numb and, if he is standing, he goes down on his knees. The heart starts beating at a terrible speed and his respiration is very rapid. Then he feels as if he were ascending into the cosmos, every fiber of his body trembling with happiness."

This experience, called the "rush," and often explicitly likened to a total body orgasm, is a highly prized and psychologically potent effect that often profoundly affects much of a user's subsequent pattern of drug use. This occurs, first, because the effect becomes autonomously desired (i.e., over and above the stimulant effects that persist after the rush abates). This predisposes to repeated injections (or, with cocaine base, smoking) and a cyclic "binge" pattern of use. Second, as shown by Jonsson et al. (29), rushes are dose-dependent. Thus, larger doses may be taken at a time when an oral user might judge that he or she has had enough. Finally, the profoundly reinforcing effects seem to induce a proportionately severe degree of dependence. Most investigators concur on this point. Kalant (30) explicitly noted that "the rate and strength of development of psychological dependence was intensified by intravenous use." Both Siegel (57) and Van Dyke and Byck (63) have stressed the importance of smoking and injection as a determinant of severe cocaine dependence. Siegel (58) has more recently reported a 9-year follow-up study of initially recreational cocaine users in which all of those who became uncontrolled, compulsive users had been inhaling cocaine base. Our own observations are anecdotal, but we certainly have noted that dependence is usually more severe and refractory in intravenous stimulant abusers.

Tolerance

Tolerance to effects of CNS stimulants has been rather extensively studied in animals and is known to develop to some effects (anorexia, hyperthermia, increased urinary excretion of catecholamines, and lethality) but not to others, such as increased locomotor activity and stereotyped behavior (35). The mechanism of this tolerance appears not to be metabolic. Studies in both animals (34,35) and humans (1) show similar half-lives (of amphetamine) in tolerant and naive animals (or volunteers).

A possible mechanism for tolerance to the noradrenergic effects of amphetamine that has been proposed is the accumulation of the amphetamine metabolite parahydroxynorephedrine as a false transmitter (12). However, it has been shown that this mechanism cannot explain all aspects of amphetamine tolerance because (a) this mechanism of tolerance was found to apply to male but not female rats (56); (b) the rate of tolerance development does not parallel accumulation of the false transmitter (34,37); (c) tolerance occurs to the hyperthermic effect of *l*-amphetamine (37) which is not a substrate for dopamine b hydroxylase and which therefore is not converted to the false transmitter; and (d) such tolerance also occurs after chronic *d*-amphetamine administration in the guinea pig, a species that does not metabolize amphetamine by parahydroxylation and therefore does not produce parahydroxynorephedrine (55).

The neurochemical correlates of tolerance (to amphetamine and phenmetrazine) have been studied in several animal species (36). The findings were complex and will not be reviewed in detail here. For example, species differences occurred, and although the effects of phenmetrazine on brain catecholamines differed from those of amphetamine, cross-tolerance between the two agents was shown.

In humans, tolerance is generally thought to occur to anorectic and cardiovascular effects of CNS stimulants, since weight loss stops after several weeks of their administration and massive doses of stimulants are often taken by abusers without lethality. Connell (15), for example, documented only very mild blood pressure elevations even after high doses were taken. Although in general this probably is true, both concepts can be criticized. For example, although weight loss diminishes and finally ceases while stimulants are taken chronically, stopping their administration in some cases leads to gains of weight, suggesting some persistant tonic effects. As to effects on blood pressure, some subjects in our challenge studies showed virtually no effects on blood pressure even after a first exposure to *d*-amphetamine at a dose of 0.5 mg/kg. Had such individuals been seen after chronic use, tolerance surely would have been assumed.

A type of tolerance to CNS stimulants that clearly does occur clinically is an acute tolerance after a single dose (20), which disappears quickly (48). This effect demonstrated by Fischman et al. (20) probably is clinically meaningful during the course of an individual stimulant binge and could either contribute to abusers' safety or, conversely, lead to higher doses being taken. Fischman et al. (20) pretreated subjects with intranasal (IN) cocaine, 96 mg. As a placebo, cocaine itself was used in a dose previously shown to have no cardiovascular or subjective effects. An hour later subjects received randomized injections of saline placebo, 16, 32, or 48 mg cocaine. The cocaine-pretreated subjects showed dramatic decrements of the effects of intravenous cocaine as compared to the placebo-pretreated subjects.

To date, this pattern of acute tolerance has been shown only with cocaine, but pharmacokinetic studies of single doses of amphetamine at our center (B. Angrist et al., *in preparation*) clearly show decrements of the effects of oral *d*-amphetamine at a time when plasma levels have plateaued rather than declined. A similar dissociation between euphoria and plasma levels occurs after single doses of cocaine (IN or inhaled) (63). We therefore think that such data may reflect a similar phenomenon and probably indicate depletion of levels of neurotransmitters released by both cocaine and amphetamine, although other mechanisms, such as acute receptor desensitization and diffusion of drug from brain into plasma might well also be factors in this dissociation between plasma level and response (63).

Supersensitivity

Augmentation of responses to CNS stimulants over time or the development of increasingly pathological responses has been reported in at least 20 preclinical studies to date (and perhaps twice that number). This sensitization has most frequently been observed in studies of the motoric effects of CNS stimulants such as locomotor activity, stereotypy, and induction of dyskinesias (43) and is indeed a robust and consistent preclinical finding. This body of literature has recently been reviewed most thoughtfully by Post and Contel (43), who emphasized that although such sensitization has been observed frequently, its occurrence can be exquisitely sensitive to a variety of variables, such as age, sex, species, dosage regimen, genetics, and conditioning effects. Thus, there do appear to be complex determinants to this frequently observed finding.

Comments on Clinical Significance of Tolerance and Supersensitivity

In the face of all of the above, this review will express the (perhaps heretical) position that in human studies the evidence for clinically meaningful tolerance or supersensitivity is scanty. Narcoleptics usually do not have to substantially increase or decrease the dose of stimulant drug that they take over time, and abusers generally report rather consistent relationships between dosage taken and effects experienced (63).

It has been proposed that the stimulant psychoses may particularly be mediated by such sensitization. Although stimulant psychoses are certainly most frequently seen in chronic abusers, they also frequently occur when doses greater than accustomed ones are taken. Furthermore, most abusers do not start using CNS stimulants at high doses, and the late occurrence of psychoses might simply reflect the time taken for escalation of dosage above a psychotogenic threshold. Conversely, the occurrence of stimulant psychoses after single large doses of stimulant agents in naive or relatively naive subjects is well documented. Of Connell's 42 cases, 8 fell into this category. None of these were considered addicts (15). Kalant (30) collected 54 cases of acute and subacute amphetamine intoxication, 30 of whom showed psychotic signs and symptoms. Most of these occurred after a single dose of amphetamine, and none of these had used the drug for over a month (30).

Pharmacological studies of chronic stimulant administration frequently open with the observation that schizophreniform psychoses are often observed after chronic CNS stimulant abuse. This implies that such psychoses do not occur in the context of acute use. This is clearly not the case. While chronicity of exposure may well cause sensitization and predispose to psychosis, such chronicity cannot be considered a sine qua non for psychotic reactions.

Psychiatric Status

Schizophrenia

Schizophrenics' responses to CNS stimulants are heterogeneous and probably, in part, state-dependent (8). In an early review of the effects of amphetamine, Reifenstein and Davidoff (46) noted seven studies in which amphetamine had been administered to schizophrenic populations. In these studies, improvement, worsening, and little change in psychiatric status were all described. Modern studies have replicated this heterogeneity of response. Janowski et al. (26) and Angrist et al. (6) have emphasized the acute increase in psychotic symptoms sometimes seen after CNS stimulant administration. Kornetsky (32) observed such hyporesponsivity in a chronic population that no effects on sleep were seen even after 20 mg d-amphetamine was administered at 8 p.m.

State dependence of response to CNS stimulants was first suggested in a study in which Janowski et al. (26) performed intravenous methyphenidate challenges in thirteen schizophrenic subjects, both while actively psychotic and after remission. In these studies, psychotic symptoms increased after the challenges done during the acute phase of the illness but did not after recovery. A variety of other evidence suggesting a state dependent component in the response of schizophrenics has been reviewed by Angrist and Van Kammen (8).

Major Affective Disorders

In depression, cocaine has been shown to improve the mood of some patients, whereas, in others, cathartic tearfulness occurred (44). A similar pattern and range of effects has been seen after administration of amphetamine to depressed patients (59). In bipolar patients, mania has been precipitated by doses of amphetamine in the 15 to 20 mg range (13). High dose *l*-DOPA, which certainly also causes psychomotor stimulant effects, has also been shown to precipitate hypomania or mania rather consistantly in bipolar subjects (39).

CLINICAL EFFECTS OF CNS STIMULANTS

Euphoria

Although the available evidence suggests that the euphoria induced by these agents is dose-related (29), many individuals find dysphoric effects increasingly admixed as dose increases (see above). Abusers of CNS stimulants appear able and willing to tolerate this admixture and seldom spontaneously reduce their accustomed dosage. The intense euphoria following intravenous administration of CNS stimulants noted above has been pharmacologically dissected in a classic series of studies by Jonsson and co-workers (27,29). In an initial study, detoxified nonpsychotic amphetamine abusers rated the intensity of effects of intravenous amphetamine on a scale of 1 to 10. Doses of 20, 40, 80, and 160 mg were given, and the intensity of effects was shown to be dose-related (29). Pretreatment with α-methyl-p-tyrosine (AMPT), 6 g over 26 hr prior to rechallenge with the highest dose, reduced ratings to below those obtained after 20 mg (29). Subsequent studies, however, showed tolerance to this effect of AMPT (28). In further studies, the effects of neuroleptics and adrenergic blockers on intravenous amphetamine euphoria were assessed. Phenoxypenzamine and propranolol were without effect, whereas chronic chlorpromazine and single doses of pimozide reduced but did not completely block the euphoria induced by 200 mg *d,l*-amphetamine i.v. (27). These findings suggest at least a partial role of dopaminergic mechanisms in mediating the euphoria induced by intravenous amphetamine.

Emotionality

As noted above, moderate and moderately high doses of CNS stimulants cause emotions to become more intense and labile. This was the cause for admission in 3 of 60 patients we saw who were admitted to Bellevue Hospital after taking amphetamine. One woman, for example, cut her wrists after a rejection by a man she had just met that night (3).

In schizophrenic subjects who show increases in psychopathology after CNS stimulant challenges (6,26), affectual changes are also involved. Interestingly, these reactions can be seen as acutely occurring mirror images to the more slowly evolving therapeutic effects of neuroleptic treatment. In the latter condition, affectual indifferance to symptoms precedes their (in some cases) disappearance. In the amphetamine challenge condition, emotional responses to psychotic preoccupations or experiences become intensified and symptoms themselves then increase or appear de novo. This clinical mirror-image relationship to the neuroleptic response emphasizes the importance of dopaminergic mechanisms in mediating CNS stimulant-induced symptom intensification in schizophrenic subjects.

Withdrawal Effects

Connell (15) was probably the first to point out that depression with "definite risk of suicide" could occur after cessation of CNS stimulants. The only comment I would add is to stress that this effect is enormously variable in its severity from individual to individual. Some abusers experience only mild lethargy and demoralization after long episodes of heavy abuse. Other individuals experience such severe depression after single low doses that they abstain from CNS stimulants thereafter.

Dependence

Resnick and Schuyten-Resnick (49) found that five patterns of (general) drug use established by The National Commission on Marijuana and Drug Use could be applied to cocaine users. These patterns—experimental, recreational, circumstantial, intensified, and compulsive—have subsequently been further discussed by the same investigators (48). In brief, experimental use is short-term and non-patterned. Recreational stimulant use can be likened to social drinking. It is without deleterious physical or psychosocial effects and is characterized by an attitude of being able to take or leave the drug. The drug is rarely purchased but may be taken if offered. Circumstantial use of stimulants occurs when these agents are taken in specific circumstances only. Resnick and Resnick (48) give as an example musicians who feel they cannot perform satisfactorily without being high on cocaine or, conversely, individuals who never use the drug when working but do during leisure time. Another example might be students who use amphetamine only during examinations. Intensified use is a pattern in which an individual feels she or he needs stimulants to meet the day-to-day demands of work. Doses are usually kept small so that consciousness is not altered to a marked degree. Such individuals might take small doses of CNS stimulants orally each morning or snort small amounts of cocaine throughout the day. Compulsive use represents a very severe degree of dependence where the drug dominates the individual's life. When not obtaining or using the drug, he or she can often think of little else. Resnick and Resnick (48) describe an individual who asked to have his bank book locked up, having already spent most of his savings and knowing that he would use the rest in a few days if he had access to his funds. Khantzian (31) describes a woman who used about 2 oz ($5,000 worth) of cocaine weekly intravenously.

Very little quantitative data exists about the important issue of progression of dependence. Siegel (58) has provided data from a 9-year follow-up of 99 recreational cocaine users, in which, at the end of the 9-year period, 49 had dropped out, but of the 50 remaining, 25 (50%) remained recreational users, 16 (32%) developed circumstantial use patterns, 4 (8%) became intensified users, and 5 (10%) became compulsive users. As noted above, the compulsive group consisted entirely of cocaine-base smokers. Except for tragic consequences that occur during intoxication states and serious medical complications of stimulant abuse, compulsive dependence probably represents the most serious consequence of the abuse of this class of agents. A pharmacologic treatment for this condition would certainly be important.

In Sweden, a past attempt at maintenance prescription of stimulants to addicts was considered a failure and abandoned (11). Perhaps a small degree of cautious optimism can be taken from (B. Angrist and S. Gershon, *unpublished,* 1979) studies in which we administered high doses of pemoline to CNS stimulant abusers. These subjects did not like the effects of high-dose pemoline, reporting that it made them too jittery. Perhaps in carefully selected abusers (such as those with the intensified use pattern described above), pemoline might prove helpful. Caution, however, is warranted since a case of pemoline abuse and psychosis (in an individual predisposed to central stimulant dependence) has recently been reported (42).

Imipramine and amino acid neurotransmitter precursors have been reported to block cocaine euphoria and to ameliorate cocaine dependence (50), but controlled studies assessing this effect have not been reported to date. Desmethylimipramine (alone) was not shown to be efficacious in one placebo-controlled trial in cocaine-dependent subjects (62).

Effects on Sexuality

CNS stimulants have a reputation as aphrodisiacs, and in some individuals, this effect is said to be the main motivation for use of these drugs (48,51). This reputation comes not from the consistency of this effect but from its intensity in those predisposed to respond in this way. Thus, increased sexual feelings and some dramatic sexual behavioral effects were reported by abusers to Kramer (33), Connell (15), Bell and Trethowan (10), Ellinwood (16), Rylander (51), and Angrist and Gershon (3,5). However, in all of these reports in which quantitative data were given, it was clear that these effects were experienced only by subgroups of patients. If one (as an exercise only) combines that data reported by Bell and Trethowan, Connell, and Angrist and Gershon, one gets a number of 116 abusers seen, of whom 29 reported intensified sexual feelings and 10 reported decreased sexual feelings.

In our abusers, there was consistency of effect among individuals; i.e., the effects on sexuality experiences did seem stable over time. Finally, cocaine in particular has a reputation as an aphrodisiac, but we know of no data in which the effects of cocaine on sexual feelings have been compared to the effects of other CNS stimulants.

Stereotypy

Stereotyped behavior is characteristically seen after rather high doses of CNS stimulants are administered and occurs in both animals and humans. In animals, stereotypies become increasingly complex in higher species. Thus, rats sniff and bite, cats show either sniffing or side-to-side head turning, dogs often show sniffing or repetitive locomotor patterns, and monkeys show hand–eye stereotypies (19). Randrup and Munkvad (45) have demonstrated the importance of striatal dopaminergic hyperactivity as a substrate for these behaviors.

In humans, stereotypy may take forms such as persistent repetitive dismantling of mechanical objects, cleaning, bathing, doodling, or searching for imaginary things. Dramatic examples have been described by Rylander (51) and Schorring (53): "During a burglary one addict . . . searched hour after hour in the flat for money all the time with an increasing fear that someone would discover him" (51). "In one case a motorcycle gang was stopped by the police because they had been driving 200 times around the same block of houses" (53). Both Rylander (51) and Schorring (53) have questioned stimulant addicts about the experience of "punding" (as such stereotyped behavior is called in slang in Scandanavia). Both indicate that the experience is pleasant and excludes any social interaction. Schorring indicates that forced interruption causes anxiety or irritation (53). Rylander noted that the activity is accompanied by a novel distortion of time sense (51).

Violence

The incidence of violent behavior varies in different reports, but the occurrence of such behavior is noted in most studies of stimulant abusers. Connell (15) indicated that hostile or aggressive behavior occurred in 22% of subjects. Griffith (23) described sudden episodes of violence at amphetamine parties. Kramer (33) indicated that most high-dose amphetamine users described episodes "in which murder or mayhem was avoided by the slimmest of margins."

Perhaps it is more important to convey the quality of these acts than to try to define their exact incidence. The most detailed descriptions are given in Ellinwood's (18) discussion of 13 homicides committed while intoxicated with amphetamine. The murders ranged from the grossly psychotic—A "27-year-old truck driver shot his boss in the back of the head because he thought the boss was trying to release poison gas into the back seat of the car in which he was riding. 'I thought they had gassed me. My boss kept reaching down beside him and pulling on something. I then got up on my elbow and shot my boss, who was driving' "—to the seemingly unmotivated—"During an argument with her paramour, this 32-year-old woman pulled a pistol out of her waistband, stuck it in his stomach, and calmly fired. When the victim got out of the car, she followed him and stated, 'You wanted to die; I showed you.' She then shot the victim twice more. She turned to a bystander and said, 'Turn him over and take a picture of his pretty face.' . . . She later got in the back seat of the patrol car, propped her feet up, and tickled the sheriff on the ear, asking him if it felt good."

A similiarly bizarre quality and range of assaults was seen in our series of 60 patients hospitalized after taking amphetamine (3), although only 2 of the 60 actually became violent. One (who had been a mugger off drugs) punched people without provocation three to four times, then, frightened, came to the hospital voluntarily. He explained that he felt like "king of the universe" and that certain people "didn't belong in my picture of things, so I took them out of the picture." The second patient saw his roommate sleeping and felt that he "looked dead." He then took a detached doorknob and beat him on the head until restrained by a second roommate. Thus, one must conclude that the quality of stimulant-induced violence is such that regardless of its incidence, it is certainly of significant concern.

Temporal Lobe Epilepsy-Like Experiences

In 1967, Ellinwood (16) called attention to a characteristic and interesting group of symptoms frequently but not invariably associated with moderately high-dose stimulant use. Although not formally psychotic, the experiences often were preludes to psychotic experiences. These included a sense of a presence or of being watched, olfactory hallucinations, changes in sexuality, deja vu experiences, an acute sense of novelty or curiosity, false recognition, distortion of body image, feelings of portentousness, philosophical concerns (with "meanings, beginnings, and essences") and "Eureka" experiences. In a subsequent paper, Ellinwood (17) stressed the similarity of these symptoms to those associated with temporal lobe epilepsy and the theoretical implications of this similarity.

CNS Stimulant Psychoses

Amphetamine produces the most widely known of the stimulant psychoses. Both for this reason and because most of our direct clinical experience is with patients or subjects who have taken amphetamine, we will discuss this condition as the prototype of the CNS stimulant psychosis.

First described by Young and Scoville in 1938 (66), amphetamine psychosis was initially observed in narcoleptics for whom the drug was prescribed. Thereafter, sporadic reports of small series or single cases appeared in the medical literature, but the condition was still considered to be rather rare. In 1958, Connell's now classic monograph on amphetamine psychosis was published (15). In that report, which studied 42 patients with amphetamine psychosis, Connell concluded that "psychosis associated with amphetamine usage is more frequent than would be expected from reports in the literature." Furthermore, he asserted that the clinical features of amphetamine psychosis were such as to make it "indistinguishable from acute or chronic paranoid schizophrenia." His contention was not accepted without controversy. Slater (60), reviewing Connell's monograph, pointed out that amphetamine psychosis, unlike schizophrenia, was characterized by a "brisk emotional reaction usually in the direction of anxiety." Bell (9) also compared the two conditions, concluding that amphetamine psychosis was rather strikingly similar to schizophrenia but that the two conditions could be differentiated by the presence of thought disorder, prominent in schizophrenia and absent in amphetamine psychosis.

Our own studies of patients hospitalized after taking amphetamine tended to bear out Connell's contention that the symptomatology of amphetamine psychosis might replicate that of schizophrenia quite closely. This is exemplified by the following case histories, all of whom were shown to have had amphetamine in their urine after hospital admission:

1. An 18-year-old injected an unknown amount of amphetamine intravenously over 2 days and began to feel that the entire city was playing a game and would not tell him. He felt that everyone and everything represented one of two main forces in the world and that other people's speech and television was directed at him. He was brought to the hospital by police at his own request.

2. A 24-year-old injected an unknown amount of amphetamine intravenously, felt he was followed by Jewish policemen, heard people talking about him, saw purple shapes in passing cars, felt he could control traffic lights, had telepathic experiences, and sang in the streets that he loved people and "lived on their hate." He was brought to the hospital by police after bizarre behavior in a subway.

3. A 19-year-old took 7 15-mg d-amphetamine capsules over 14 hr. He argued with a man in a night club and left because he was frightened of him. On the street he had the idea that while he was new in New York, the man with whom he had argued had friends that he might call to "get" him. Moreover, the man he had argued with had a "flat" face, and people on the street with "flat" faces seemed particularly ominous. He went into a bar where people looked at him with sinister amusement in a way that suggested that he was to be the "star" in a play in which he would be killed for their amusement. He asked why people were looking at him and "hassling" him, and this made people look at him all the more. He left and returned to his hotel. By the time he got there he heard a gang saying they were going to torture him. He locked, then barricaded his room. He still heard the voices and retreated across the room and out on to the (fourth floor) window ledge. He still heard the voices and, knowing he couldn't retreat further, decided to "make a run for it" and burst through his hotel door with an open penknife in his hand.

However, the study of hospitalized patients has obvious limitations. Most important of which is that predrug status cannot be known. Because of these methodological limitations, Griffith et al. in 1968 (25) undertook the first experimental induction of amphetamine psychosis in nonschizophrenic volunteer subjects. This made it possible to observe amphetamine psychosis uncontaminated by the possibility of concomitant usage of other drugs or by schizophrenia that might have antedated amphetamine ingestion.

Dextroamphetamine, 5 to 10 mg, was administered hourly for as long as the subjects tolerated it. The result was a generally abrupt onset of paranoid delusions, often with cold, detached affect. Subjects thought they were being secretly photographed or discussed on TV. One felt that the entire study was subterfuge; another believed that an assassin had been hired to kill him; a third became aware of a giant oscillator placed in the ceiling to control his thoughts and the behavior of others. However, hallucinations were not reported, and no formal thought disorders were observed (24).

We replicated the experiments of Griffith et al. (24), using similar methodology but a somewhat more aggressive dosage schedule, in which up to 50 mg/hr of racemic amphetamine was administered (4).

In the first of these studies, the subject (a shy individual diagnosed as a schizoid personality) received a cumulative dose of 325 mg of racemic amphetamine over 28.75 hr. Clinical effects were as follows:

100 mg ($7\frac{3}{4}$ hr): "The other patients went to bed and the atmosphere changed. I was the center of attention. I didn't want to talk because I was afraid I'd say something and the nurses would make a report and you'd cut me off. I felt the nurse behind me and felt like I had to hide or something."

150 mg (12 hr): During the night, one patient awoke, came into the dayroom and spoke of "brainwashing." "It seemed to me she thought I was doing it to her, making her sicker with my mind and I thought there was another person involved, putting thoughts in both our minds or using my mind to cure her." Asked if he believed in telepathy, he answered, "When I'm stoned, I do, because it feels so real."

230 mg (21 hr): Smells a "vile" smell, which he believes is caused by amphetamine being excreted in his perspiration. Feels others notice the smell. This recurs constantly during the remainder of the study, especially when he has to be close to others, that is, when his blood pressure is being taken. Initially, this is an idea, but increasingly it becomes an actual perception, causing him to take showers.

235 mg (22 hr): After lunch, he was told to lie down by an aide. He didn't want to, but did so "to avoid an argument." Lying down he "felt sure" that the investigator had "sneakily" cut his medications by substituting placebo tablets and that the amphetamine was again being excreted in his perspiration, causing a strong body odor that he actually smelled. At this time, he heard voices of other patients in the ward discussing him in the third person, i.e., "He's stupid. Why is he doing it? He's not doing anything. He's just staying up."

280 mg (26 hr): Afraid to leave the ward for a taped interview because "other people look at you and seem to know." He also smelled feces and thought he had been incontinent but checked and found none.

325 mg (28.75 hr): Taking his temperature in the bathroom, he noticed someone in the lab across the street and felt that he had been "planted" there to watch him.

Thus, from the onset in these studies, we were able to document hallucinatory phenomena (olfactory and auditory).

The presence or absence of thought disorder in amphetamine psychosis is controversial. We thought, in this study, that the subject did show some mild dose-related disturbance of thought. Although grossly autistic productions were not encountered, he became progressively irrelevant and diffuse. (In another subject, this same type of thinking disturbance was more dramatic. When asked how he felt, after 430 mg *l*-amphetamine, he answered, "agitated and annoyed." Asked why, he responded: "It's a ridiculous thing, like the marijuana laws or birth control. That's totally ridiculous! Just like a thunderstorm in the forest. It affects young trees. There is a balance of nature. You mess with the balance of nature, you lose buffalo, you lose birds. Things become extinct. For man, you lose philosophies.") (2)

A third subject showed a much more dramatic pattern of thought disorganization. After receiving 595 mg of racemic amphetamine, he spoke in a quite disorganized and bizarre way. He felt that he had become "a prophet" who was being addressed directly by God and first wrote his "relevations" frantically and then "preached" them loudly to the ward at large: "My consciousness in the form of what you know as human. My feeling which I receive from Him. I bring the answer to the unknown and yet. They who do not hear or show, laugh or murder my love. In my human form, He might let me act human, for the rest must still wonder at my actions, which make them doubt my having been used to enlighten. Every thought that stops me from accepting all knowledge, more than man has ever known. It is just part of the supreme game to make you wait until it is time for you to receive everlasting good. It is not mine to give. I am His, I bring His will, call it prophet" (2,4). His written productions are shown in Fig. 1.

However, other subjects experienced reactions in which thought content was grossly psychotic, yet form remained quite intact. One, for example, after 465 mg racemic amphetamine over 23 hr, experienced an acute and florid paranoid hallucinatory psychosis. He first saw "colored haloes" around lights, then "heard" a gang coming on the ward to kill him. His paranoid feelings extended to the experimenter who, he assumed, had "set up the trap." At times, he was quite hostile. Explanations that his experiences were drug-induced were rejected with sardonic mock agreement (e.g., "Oh sure! Hah! Is that the way it's going to be?"). At other times, he would become tearful and beg the experimenter to explain "what was really going on." He had visual hallucinations of gangsters and doors opening and closing in the shadows, and visual illusions (e.g., paper on a bulletin

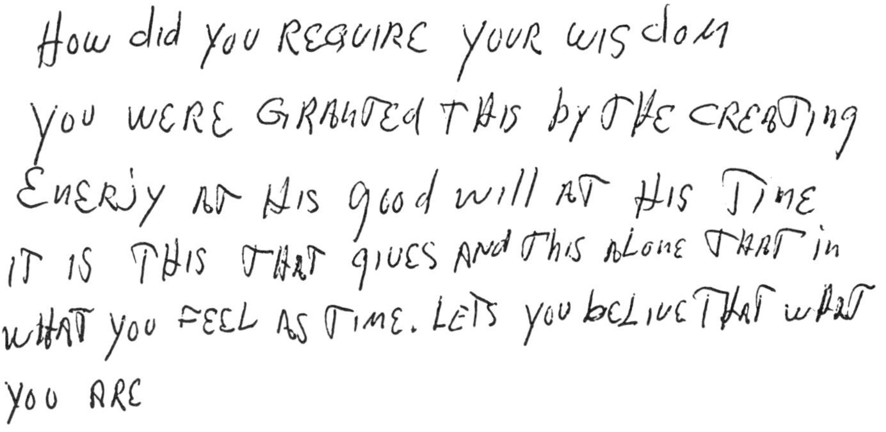

How did you REQUIRE your wisdom

you WERE GRANTED THIS by THE CREATing

EnERJy AT His good will AT His Time

IT IS THIS THAT gives And This aLone THAT in

wHAT you FEEL AS Time. LETS you beLive THAT wHAT

you ARE

FIG. 1. Written productions of a nonpsychotic subject who received 590 mg racemic amphetamine over 46 hr. Writing done after 575 mg.

board "turned into" a gangster in a white raincoat). He jumped at the slightest sound, assuming it was the gang coming to "get" him, and was so frightened that he refused to investigate the ward to "prove" that no one was really there. When the gang was not "heard" or "seen," he constantly "sensed their presence." He was certain that the end point of the experiment was for him to be killed (2).

On the basis of these studies, we concluded that Connell's opinion that amphetamine psychosis "may be indistinguishable from acute or chronic paranoid schizophrenia" had been corroborated.

CNS Stimulants as Clinical Research Tools in Schizophrenia

This area has rather recently been reviewed (8). Rather than repeat (or attempt to summarize) that material, I would like to briefly describe a new study at our center (A. Wolkin et al., *in preparation*) in which the effects of amphetamine on local cerebral glucose metabolism of schizophrenic and nonschizophrenic subjects were assessed. A total of 16 schizophrenic subjects and 6 normal controls received placebo before a [^{11}C]deoxyglucose PET scan in the morning. After the scan, 10 schizophrenic subjects and all 8 controls received 0.5 mg/kg d-amphetamine by mouth. Of the schizophrenic subjects, 6 received placebo at this time. A second scan was done 2 hr after the second set of capsules.

A generalized morning-to-afternoon increase in glucose metabolism was seen in the 6 placebo-treated schizophrenic subjects. (A separately studied group of about 20 normal controls, scanned similarly in morning and afternoon, but without placebo-capsules, showed small morning-to-afternoon increases.)

By contrast, amphetamine-treated schizophrenics and (even more) amphetamine-treated controls showed decreases of cerebral glucose metabolism (Fig. 2), which correlated with plasma amphetamine levels drawn at the time of the second scan (Fig. 3).

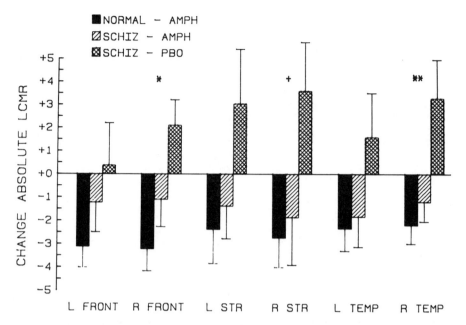

FIG. 2. Effects of amphetamine 0.5 mg/kg on local cerebral metabolic rates (LCMR), expressed as micromoles of glucose/100 g tissue/min in 10 schizophrenic subjects and 8 controls. The effects of placebo on LCMR of 6 schizophrenic subjects is also shown. $\dagger p < 0.10$; $*p < 0.05$; $**p < 0.01$; ANOVA.

Wolkin et al. (65) had previously shown that chronic neuroleptic treatment increased glucose metabolism in schizophrenics and that this increase was less brisk in frontal regions than other brain areas. These new data in which amphetamine decreased metabolism therefore are pharmacologically consistent. Furthermore, the amphetamine-induced decreases in metabolism were also

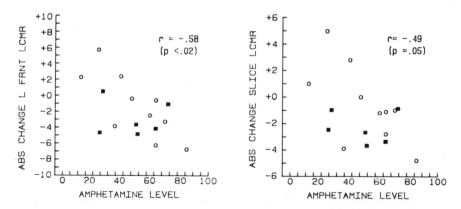

FIG. 3. Changes in **(A)** left frontal and **(B)** whole (mid-ventricular) slice cerebral metabolic rates correlated with plasma amphetamine levels drawn immediately prior to second PET scan. *Open circle*, amphetamine-treated schizophrenics; *filled square*, amphetamine-treated controls.

muted in frontal areas in schizophrenic subjects and were less than the decreases shown by controls (Fig. 2). Thus, from these two studies, some consistency emerges regarding the effects of dopamine agonists and antagonists on cerebral glucose metabolism. Moreover, the concept of a frontal lobe locus for aberrant brain function in schizophrenics (25a,25b,64) is supported.

REFERENCES

1. Anggard, E., Jonsson, L. E., Hogmark, A. L., and Gunne, L. M. (1973): Amphetamine metabolism in amphetamine psychosis. *Clin. Pharmacol. Ther.,* 14:870–880.
2. Angrist, B. (1983): Psychoses induced by central nervous system stimulants and related drugs. In: *Stimulants: Neurochemical, Behavioral and Clinical Perspectives,* edited by I. Creese, pp. 1–30. Raven Press, New York.
3. Angrist, B., and Gershon, S. (1969): Amphetamine abuse in New York City—1966 to 1968. *Seminars in Psychiatry,* 1:195–207.
4. Angrist, B., and Gershon, S. (1970): The phenomenology of experimentally induced amphetamine psychosis. Preliminary observations. *Biol. Psychiatry,* 2:95–107.
5. Angrist, B., and Gershon, S. (1976): Clinical effects of amphetamine and l-DOPA on sexuality and aggression. *Compr. Psychiatry,* 17:715–722.
6. Angrist, B., Rotrosen, J., and Gershon, S. (1980): Response to apomorphine, amphetamine and neuroleptics in schizophrenic subjects. *Psychopharmacology (Berlin),* 67:31–38.
7. Angrist, B., and Sudilovsky, A. (1978): Central nervous system stimulants: Historical aspects and clinical effects. In: *Handbook of Psychopharmacology, Vol. 11,* edited by L. L. Iversen, S. D. Iversen, and S. H. Snyder, pp. 99–165. Plenum Press, New York.
8. Angrist, B., and van Kammen, D. (1984): CNS stimulants as tools in the study of schizophrenia. *Trends in Neurosciences,* 7:388–390.
9. Bell, D. S. (1965): A comparison of amphetamine psychosis and schizophrenia. *Br. J. Psychiatry,* 3:701–706.
10. Bell, D. S., and Trethowan, W. H. (1961): Amphetamine addiction and disturbed sexuality. *Arch. Gen. Psychiatry,* 4:74–78.
11. Bergsman, A., and Jarpe, G. (1969): Comments on free prescription of central stimulants and narcotic drugs. In: *Abuse of Central Stimulants,* edited by F. Sjoqvist and M. Tottie, pp. 275–277. Almqvist and Wiksell, Stockholm.
12. Brodie, B. B., Cho, A. K., and Gessa, G. L. (1970): Possible role of p-hydroxynorephedrine in the depletion of norepinephrine induced by d-amphetamine and in tolerance to this drug. In: *International Symposium on Amphetamine and Related Compounds,* edited by E. Costa and S. Garrattine, pp. 217–230. Raven Press, New York.
13. Bunney, W. E., Jr. (1978): Psychopharmacology of the switch process in affective illness. In: *Psychopharmacology: A Generation of Progress,* edited by M. A. Lipton, A. DiMascio, and K. F. Killam, pp. 1249–1259. Raven Press, New York.
14. Ciaranello, R. D., Barchas, R., Kessler, S., and Barchas, J. D. (1972): Catecholamines: Strain differences in biosynthetic enzyme activity in mice. *Life Sci.,* 11:565–572.
15. Connell, P. H. (1958): *Amphetamine Psychosis. Maudsley Monographs No. 5.* Oxford University Press, London.
16. Ellinwood, E. H., Jr. (1967): Amphetamine psychosis I: Description of the individuals and the process. *J. Nerv. Ment. Dis.,* 144:273–283.
17. Ellinwood, E. H., Jr. (1968): Amphetamine psychosis II: Theoretical implications. *Journal of Neuropsychiatry,* 4:45–54.
18. Ellinwood, E. H., Jr. (1971): Assault and homicide associated with amphetamine abuse. *Am. J. Psychiatry,* 127:1170–1175.
19. Ellinwood, E. H., Jr., and Sudelovsky, A. (1973): Chronic amphetamine intoxication: Behavioral model of psychosis. In: *Psychopathology and Psychopharmacology,* edited by J. O. Cole, M. Freedman, and A. J. Friedhoff, pp. 51–70. The Johns Hopkins University Press, Baltimore.
20. Fischman, M., Schuster, C., Javaid, J., Hatano, Y., and Davis, J. (1985): Acute tolerance development to the cardiovascular and subjective effects of cocaine. *J. Pharmacol. Exp. Ther.,* 235:677–682.

21. Freud, S. (1887): Bemerkungen uber Cocainsucht und Cocainfurcht mit Beziehung auf einem Vortrag. *Wien. Med. Wochenschr.,* 28:929–932.
22. Garrattini, S., Jori, A., and Samanin, R. (1976): Interactions of various drugs with amphetamine. *Ann. N.Y. Acad. Sci.,* 281:409–425.
23. Griffith, J. (1966): A study of illicit amphetamine drug traffic in Oklahoma City. *Am. J. Psychiatry,* 123:560–569.
24. Griffith, J. D., Cavanaugh, J., Held, J., and Oates, J. A. (1972): Dextroamphetamine evaluation of psychomimetic properties in man. *Arch. Gen. Psychiatry,* 26:97–100.
25. Griffith, J. D., Oates, J., and Cavanaugh, J. (1968): Paranoid episodes induced by drug. *J.A.M.A.,* 205:39.
25a. Ingvar, D. H., and Franzen, G. (1974): Abnormalities of cerebral blood flow distribution in patients with chronic schizophrenia. *Acta Psychiat. Scand.,* 50:425–462.
25b. Ingvar, D. H., and Franzen, G. (1974): Distribution of cerebral activity in chronic schizophrenia. *The Lancet,* 2:1484–1486.
26. Janowsky, D. S., El-Yousef, M. K., Davis, J. M., and Sekerke, H. S. (1973): Provocation of schizophrenic symptoms by intravenous administration of methylphenidate. *Arch. Gen. Psychiatry,* 28:185–191.
27. Jonsson, L. E. (1972): Pharmacological blockade of amphetamine effects in amphetamine dependent subjects. *Eur. J. Clin. Pharmacol.,* 4:206–211.
28. Jonsson, L. E., Anggard, E., and Gunne, L. M. (1971): Blockade of intravenous amphetamine euphoria in man. *Clin. Pharmacol. Ther.,* 12:889–896.
29. Jonsson, L. E., Gunne, L. M., and Anggard, E. (1969): Effects of alpha-methyltyrosine in amphetamine dependent subjects. *Pharmacologia Clinica,* 2:27–29.
30. Kalant, O. J. (1973): *The Amphetamines, Toxcity and Addiction, Second Edition. Brookside Monographs of the Addiction Research Foundation No. 5.* University of Toronto Press, Toronto.
31. Khantzian, E. J. (1983): An extreme case of cocaine dependence and marked improvement with methyphenidate treatment. *Am. J. Psychiatry,* 140:784–785.
32. Kornetsky, C. (1976): Hyporesponsivity of chronic schizophrenic patients to dextroamphetamine. *Arch. Gen. Psychiatry,* 33:1425–1428.
33. Kramer, J. C. (1969): Introduction to amphetamine abuse. *Journal of Psychedelic Drugs,* 2:1–16.
34. Kuhn, C. M., and Schanberg, S. (1977): Distribution and metabolism of amphetamine in tolerant animals. In: *Cocaine and Other Stimulants,* edited by E. H. Ellinwood and M. Kilby, pp. 161–177. Plenum Press, New York and London.
35. Lewander, T. (1972): Experimental and clinical studies on amphetamine dependence. In: *Biochemical and Pharmacological Aspects of Dependence and Reports on Marijuana Research,* edited by H. M. Van Praag, pp. 69–84. De Erven F. Boun N. V., Haarlem, Netherlands.
36. Lewander, T. (1974): Effect of chronic treatment with central stimulants on brain monoamines and some behavioral and physiological functions in rats, guinea pigs and rabbits. In: *Neuropsychopharmacology of Monamines and Their Regulatory Enzymes,* edited by E. Usdin, pp. 221–239. Raven Press, New York.
37. Lewander, T., Molliis, G., and Brus, I. (1975): Mechanisms of tolerance to the hyperthermic effect of d- and l-amphetamine in rats. In: *Neuropsychopharmacology,* edited by J. R. Boissier, H. Hippius, and P. Pichot, pp. 323–334. Exerpta Medica Press, Amsterdam.
38. Maas, J. W. (1962): Neurochemical differences between two strains of mice. *Science,* 137:621–662.
39. Murphy, D. L. (1972): l-DOPA, behavioral activation and psychopathology. In: *Neurotransmitters,* edited by I. J. Kopin, pp. 472–492. Williams and Williams, Baltimore.
40. Nurnberger, J., Gershon, E., Jimerson, D., Buchsbaum, M., Gold, P., Brown, G., and Ebert, M. C. (1981): Pharmacogenetics of d-amphetamine in man. In: *Genetic Research Strategies for Psychobiology and Psychiatry,* edited by E. S. Gershon, S. Matthysse, X. O. Breakfield, and R. D. Ciaranello, pp. 257–268. Boxwood Press, Pacific Grove, California.
41. Pickens, R., Thompson, T., and Yokel, R. A. (1972): Characteristics of amphetamine self administration by rats. In: *Current Concepts of Amphetamine Abuse* (publication No. HSM 72-9085), edited by E. H. Ellinwood, Jr. and S. Cohen, pp. 43–48. Department of Health, Education and Welfare; U.S. Government Printing Office, Washington, D.C.
42. Polchert, S. E., and Morse, R. M. (1985): Pemoline abuse. *J.A.M.A.,* 254:946–947.
43. Post, R. M., and Contel, N. P. (1983): Human and animal studies of cocaine: Implications for development of behavioral pathology. In: *Stimulants: Neurochemical, Behavioral and Clinical Perspectives,* edited by I. Creese, pp. 169–203. Raven Press, New York.

44. Post, R. M., Kotin, J., and Goodwin, F. K. (1974): The effects of cocaine on depressed patients. *Am. J. Psychiatry,* 131:511–517.
45. Randrup, A., and Munkvad, I. (1970): Biochemical, anatomical and psychological investigation of stereotyped behavior induced by amphetamines. In: *International Symposium on Amphetamines and Related Compounds,* edited by E. Costa and S. Garattini, pp. 695–713. Raven Press, New York.
46. Reifenstein, E. C., Jr., and Davidoff, E. (1939): Benzedrine sulfate therapy, the present status. *N.Y. State J. Med.,* 39:42–57.
47. Reis, D. S., Baker, H., Fink, J. S., and Joh, T. H. (1978): A genetic control of central dopamine neurons in relation to brain organization, drug responses and behavior. In: *Catecholamines: Basic and Clinical Frontiers, Vol. 1,* edited by E. Usdin, I. J. Kopin, and J. Barchas, pp. 23–33. Pergamon Press, New York.
48. Resnick, R., and Resnick, E. (1984): Cocaine abuse and its treatment. *Psychiatr. Clin. North Am.,* 7:713–728.
49. Resnick, R. B., and Schuyten-Resnick, E. (1976): Clinical aspects of cocaine: Assessment of cocaine abuse behavior in man. In: *Cocaine: Chemical, Biological, Clinical, Social and Treatment Aspects,* edited by S. J. Mule, pp. 219–228. CRC Press, Cleveland.
50. Rosecan, J. S. (1983): *The Treatment of Cocaine Abuse with Imipramine, L-Tyrosine and L-Tryptophan.* Paper presented at the VII World Congress of Psychiatry, Vienna, July 14–19.
51. Rylander, G. (1969): Clinical and medico-criminological aspects of addiction to central stimulating drugs. In: *Abuse of Control Stimulants,* edited by F. Sjoqvist and M. Tottie, pp. 251–273. Almqvist and Wiksell, Stockholm.
52. Schlesinger, K., Boggan, W., and Freedman, D. X. (1965): Genetics of audiogenic seizures: I: Relation to brain serotonin and norepinepherine in mice. *Life Sci.,* 4:2345–2351.
53. Schorring, E. (1977): Changes in individual and social behavior induced by amphetamine and related compounds in monkeys and man. In: *Cocaine and Other Stimulants,* edited by E. H. Ellinwood, Jr. and M. Kilbey, pp. 481–522. Plenum Press, New York and London.
54. Schuster, C. R., Woods, J. H., and Seevers, M. H. (1969): Self-administration of central stimulants by the monkey. In: *Abuse of Central Stimulants,* edited by F. Sjoqvist and M. Tottie, pp. 339–347. Almqvist and Wiksell, Stockholm.
55. Sever, P., and Caldwell, J. (1974): Species differences in amphetamine tolerance. *J. Pharmacol.,* 5(Suppl. 2):91.
56. Sever, P. S., Caldwell, J., and Williams, R. T. (1974): Evidence against the involvement of false transmitters in tolerance to amphetamine-induced hyperthermia in the rat. *J. Pharm. Pharmacol.,* 26:823–826.
57. Siegel, R. K. (1979): Cocaine smoking. *N. Engl. J. Med.,* 300:373.
58. Siegel, R. K. (1984): Changing patterns of cocaine use: Longitudinal observations, consequences, and treatment. In: *Cocaine: Pharmacology, Effects and Treatment of Abuse (NIDA Research Monograph #50)* (Publication no. ADM 84-1326), edited by J. Grabowski, pp. 92–110. United States Department of Health and Human Services; U.S. Government Printing Office, Washington, D.C.
59. Silberman, E. K., Reus, V. I., Jimerson, D. C., Lynott, A. M., and Post, R. M. (1981): Heterogeneity of amphetamine response in depressed patients. *Am. J. Psychiatry,* 138:1302–1307.
60. Slater, E. (1959): Review of amphetamine psychosis by P. H. Connell. *Br. Med. J.,* 1:488.
61. Sudak, H. S., and Maas, J. (1964): Central nervous system serotonin and norepinephrine localization in emotional and non-emotional strains in mice. *Nature,* 203:1255–1256.
62. Tennant, F. S., and Rawson, R. A. (1983): Cocaine and amphetamine dependence treated with desipramine. In: *Problems of Drug Dependence (NIDA Research Monograph #43)* (Publication no. ADM 83-1264), United States Dept. of Health and Human Services; U.S. Government Printing Office, Washington, D.C.
63. Van Dyke, C., and Byck, R. (1982): Cocaine. *Sci. Am.,* 246:128–141.
64. Weinberger, D. R., Berman, K. F., and Zec, R. F. (1986): Physiological dysfunction of dorsolateral prefrontal cortex in schizophrenia: I. Regional cerebral blood flow evidence. *Arch. Gen. Psychiatry,* 43:114–124.
65. Wolkin, A., Jaeger, J., Brodie, J. D., Wolf, A., Fowler, J., Rotrosen, J., Gomez-Mont, F., and Cancro, R. (1985): Persistance of cerebral metabolic abnormalities in chronic schizophrenia as detected by positron emission tomography. *Am. J. Psychiatry,* 142:564–571.
66. Young, D., and Scoville, W. B. (1938): Paranoid psychosis in narcolepsy and the possible danger of benzedrine treatment. *Med. Clin. North Am.,* 22:637–646.

Brain Reward Systems and Abuse, edited by
J. Engel and L. Oreland.
Raven Press, New York © 1987.

Strategies for the Identification and Testing of New Pharmacological Modulators of Ethanol Consumption

Claudio A. Naranjo, John T. Sullivan, Mary O. Lawrin, and Edward M. Sellers

Clinical Pharmacology Program, Addiction Research Foundation Clinical Institute, and Departments of Pharmacology and Medicine, University of Toronto, Toronto, Ontario M5S 2S1, Canada

Alcoholism and alcohol-related problems occur in approximately 20% of the adult population (56). Pharmacotherapies can be useful therapeutic interventions when used alone or in conjunction with psychosocial treatments in individuals who have medical and/or psychosocial problems related to excessive alcohol consumption. The aims of pharmacotherapies intended to attenuate drinking are (a) to decrease the frequency and/or severity of alcohol-induced organic diseases such as alcoholic liver disease and/or (b) to attenuate or prevent the many psychosocial problems that these individuals develop.

A number of previous reviews (38,44,53) have commented on the lack of effective drugs for reducing alcohol consumption. The most commonly prescribed agents still are the alcohol-sensitizing drugs (e.g., disulfiram), which, when given prior to alcohol, induce an aversive physiological reaction that is supposed to deter further drinking. However, the very few randomized controlled trials have yielded inconclusive results about their efficacy (35,38,47). Also, these drugs have several disadvantages such as unknown optimal dose and dosage schedule, unknown therapeutic margin, several contraindications for use (e.g., liver disease), substantial and diverse drug-related toxicity, and potentially deleterious drug interactions. Further problems with this strategy include the toxicity of acetaldehyde (47) and the possible involvement of acetaldehyde in the reinforcing properties of ethanol (58). Moreover, the alcohol-sensitizing drugs can only be used when the treatment goal is abstinence (47). Thus, problem drinkers who would prefer a moderate drinking goal do not have a treatment option combining behavioral interventions and drugs.

The views expressed in this publication are those of the authors and do not necessarily reflect those of the Addiction Research Foundation.

In this review, we will analyze conceptual and methodological aspects concerning the development of new pharmacological treatments for alcohol abusers. We will frequently refer to our experiences in testing serotonin (5-HT) uptake inhibitors.

NEED FOR INNOVATION IN THE DEVELOPMENT OF DRUG TREATMENTS FOR ALCOHOLISM

Interest in new pharmacological treatments for alcoholism has slowly but steadily increased in recent years (8,29,38,40). Systematic approaches to the problem have been confined to a few groups of researchers. Several factors have retarded innovative research into the pharmacotherapy of alcoholism (44).

A major reason has been the apparent lack of interest by the pharmaceutical industry in this area (7,29,38). Pharmaceutical companies continue to spend millions of dollars to develop new anxiolytics and diuretics even though the prototype drugs (i.e., diazepam and furosemide) are very effective. Today there are more than 25 marketed benzodiazepines. Unless it can be shown that a new agent is substantially better in clinically relevant terms, it is reasonable to question the need to continue to invest in areas of research that are unlikely to result in really innovative drugs. Another consideration is that there is no relationship between research expenses and the relative size of the potential market. Alcohol-related problems are more prevalent than other conditions for which large investments are made. Also, clinical investigators usually have to use drugs, originally developed for other indications, to test their effects in alcohol abusers. We believe improvements in all these areas are possible. For example, pharmaceutical companies could begin systematic research programs to discover and clinically test new drugs for alcohol-related problems. This could provide a major impetus to further this research.

Basic and clinical researchers have shown little interest in improving the pharmacotherapy of alcoholism. Some argue that the problem is too complicated and that more can be accomplished in other research areas with the same amount of effort. This attitude is usually associated with the belief that alcoholics are hopeless individuals to whom very little can be offered. Research advances that are actively being pursued by several investigators suggest that this view is too pessimistic (40).

From a conceptual point of view, a major clinical problem is that alcoholics are considered to be a homogeneous population. Alcohol abuse is a multidimensional condition (56). The systematic assessment on three dimensions (drinking history, alcohol dependence, and associated biomedical and psychosocial problems) identifies subtypes of alcohol abusers who may respond differently to treatment. A number of studies indicate that their prevalence in a population is as follows: alcoholics (5%), problem drinkers (20%), social drinkers (60%), and abstainers (15%) (56). Therefore, it is reasonable to question whether too much attention has been paid to the 5% of classic alcoholics. Perhaps it would be appropriate to intensify the efforts for the early identification of and the early interventions for problem drinkers who have a greater chance of recovery and who represent a large proportion of the alcohol abusers (57).

DESIRABLE CHARACTERISTICS OF NEW DRUGS

New drugs for moderating alcohol intake should comply with a number of prerequisites before they can become useful therapeutic agents (44). The ideal drug should have the following properties: (a) Application of an active dose of the drug should produce a consistent and robust effect in the responders. This would help to develop appropriate expectations of success. (b) The active dose of the drug should not have deleterious interactions with ethanol that could interfere with everyday life. (c) The drug should be easily administered to subjects (e.g., oral route), and the procedure should encourage compliance with treatment. (d) The drug should be long-acting, in order to simplify its administration and possibly enhance compliance. (e) The agent should preferentially be capable of antagonizing some of the deleterious effects of ethanol (e.g., memory impairment, impaired psychomotor performance) in addition to attenuating ethanol intake. This property might also help to convince the individual that attenuation of drinking will be associated with some improvement of performance in other areas. (f) The drug should have a wide therapeutic margin, which would prevent serious reactions in the case of an eventual overdose. (g) It should be reasonably safe, and the side effects of the drug should not significantly affect subjects' functioning (e.g., motor skills). In addition, the agent should not further accentuate any of the mechanisms by which ethanol induces organic damage (e.g., increase acetaldehyde concentration).

STRATEGIES FOR THE IDENTIFICATION AND TESTING OF NEW PHARMACOLOGICAL MODULATORS OF ETHANOL INTAKE

A research program for the identification and testing of new drugs with some or all of the properties listed above was initiated by our group some years ago (38). The task has not been an easy one, and in this chapter we make an attempt to illustrate the challenges and opportunities we faced in our studies with serotonergic drugs.

Biological Mechanisms Regulating Ethanol Intake

The development of new pharmacologic treatments depends on our understanding of the biological mechanisms regulating ethanol intake. Recent studies suggest that a complex interaction of neurobiological and systemic factors regulate ethanol intake. Several neurotransmitters (monoamines and neuropeptides), hormones, and other factors are possibly involved in mediating the initiation, maintenance, and cessation of alcohol drinking (41). The factors mediating the initiation of ethanol intake are usually associated with the neurobiological correlates of the positive and negative reinforcement afforded by ethanol. In order to produce a positive reinforcing effect, ethanol interacts with the neurobiological substrates of reward (6). Neurotransmitters, such as norepinephrine (2) and dopamine (25), acetaldehyde (58), and several neuropeptides (18) have been postulated to mediate these effects. Ethanol exerts its negative reinforcing effects by attenuating an unpleasant or harmful state. For example, ethanol induces relaxation, promotes sleep, or relieves social or physical discomforts.

The positive and negative reinforcing properties of ethanol are necessary but not sufficient conditions to maintain excessive ethanol intake. Other factors most likely involved include the biological correlates of the development of tolerance to ethanol effects. The effects of ethanol on learning mechanisms (which may influence the abilities to remember pleasant experiences and to forget unpleasant ones) and the neurobiological correlates of the alcohol dependence syndrome may also account for the maintenance of excessive ethanol intake.

A normal individual can easily discontinue ethanol intake, but a physically dependent alcoholic usually does not have such an ability. Biological mechanisms are involved in the cessation of drinking and thereby provide the feedback necessary to discontinue further drinking. The cessation mechanisms are possibly associated with the correlates of alcohol intoxication and may involve effects such as drowsiness, impaired balance or reasoning, and adverse symptoms such as nausea or vomiting. Also, genetic variations in ethanol and acetaldehyde metabolism may play a role. Oriental subjects have a high frequency of an acetaldehyde-mediated aversive reaction to ethanol due to an acetaldehyde dehydrogenase deficiency (30). This is an example of an exaggeration of the cessation mechanisms.

Problem drinking can then be conceptualized as a disorder of the mechanisms which regulate the initiation or maintenance of drinking or as a disorder of the mechanisms which are responsible for the cessation of drinking. The elucidation of the physiological and biochemical (e.g., neurobiological, humoral, etc.) correlates of these mechanisms can eventually lead to the development of pharmacological interventions that can be used for therapeutic purposes. Since alcohol is a drug and since the organism has experienced adaptational changes to its presence, the mechanisms involved in the initiation, maintenance, or cessation of ethanol drinking most likely also subserve other functions. In addition, since ethanol apparently does not have any specific receptors in the brain, it is unrealistic to expect the development of completely selective pharmacotherapies. What matters from a clinical viewpoint is the relative balance of beneficial and adverse effects.

The identification and testing of new drugs for decreasing ethanol intake depends on the conduct of appropriate animal and human studies as described below.

Preclinical Studies

Use of Animal Models of Alcohol Consumption

At the preclinical phase of drug development, animal models provide the most obvious means of testing new drugs. A number of procedures have been developed, most of which involve oral ingestion of alcohol solutions by rats. The criteria for an adequate animal model have been suggested by Lester and Freed (24). These are (a) oral ingestion of alcohol without food deprivation; (b) substantial ingestion of alcohol with competing fluids available; (c) ingestion directed to the central intoxication character of alcohol, substantiated by determination of circulating blood alcohol levels; (d) work performed, even in the face of aversive consequences, to obtain alcohol; (e) intoxication sustained over a long period; (f) production of a withdrawal syndrome and physical dependence; and (g) after abstinence, reacquisition of drinking to intoxication and reproducibility of the alcohol process.

These criteria and several recent modifications along similar lines (e.g., ref. 4) are not necessarily valid for testing of new drugs (6,36). For example, the criteria do not take into account the clinical spectrum of alcohol-related problems (36,56). Moreover, these criteria place too much emphasis on drinking to the point of physical dependence, to the exclusion of levels of drinking that may be analogous to problem drinking in humans but do not involve physical dependence. However, the most serious limitation of these criteria is the lack of cross-validation of the model by comparing results in animals and in humans (36). This is essential, because frequently the potential clinical relevance of findings is extrapolated from results exclusively obtained in animal studies.

To our knowledge, no systematic programs have been developed by pharmaceutical companies to study drug effects on alcohol consumption (36). This work has remained mostly in the hands of academics. We recommend that some pharmaceutical companies incorporate, among their general screening batteries, a search for compounds that could decrease alcohol consumption. Our studies with 5-HT uptake inhibitors illustrate that this could be a potentially fruitful area, but without systematic procedures, the identification of useful drugs will continue to depend exclusively on the serendipitous observations of astute clinicians or researchers.

Clinical Studies for Testing New Pharmacological Modulators of Ethanol Intake

The lack of drugs specifically developed for modulating ethanol intake has originated a series of challenges in our studies. For example, we usually must use drugs that have been designed for other indications (e.g., antidepressants). This immediately creates two major problems: first, the selection of doses to be tested in alcohol abusers, and, second, the fact that we require some information about the interactions of ethanol and the drug. Usually some information is available for the latter, but with respect to the dose we can only make an educated guess. In addition, we must show that the effect we detect is independent of the presumed major therapeutic action of the drug. We have already mentioned the importance of an adequate clinical characterization of alcohol abusers, because they may respond differently to various treatments.

In subsequent sections, we will review the various phases involved in the evaluation of drug treatments. We will also consider factors that we have found to be important in studies in alcohol abusers.

OUR STRATEGY FOR CLINICAL DRUG EVALUATION

The evaluation of drugs in humans is currently conducted in four phases (39).

Phase I

This consists of the first administration of a new drug to humans and usually involves only a small number of healthy volunteers. This part of the study should provide evidence of dose-related pharmacological effects and side effects in single dose and multiple dose studies over a limited time. Evidence of drug absorption, distribution, metabolism, and excretion must be provided to determine the drug pharmacokinetic profile in humans and to optimize drug use. Since no drug has yet been specifically developed for alcohol abusers, clinical investigators must use drugs developed for other indications. The information collected in Phase I trials is usually available when studies in alcohol abusers are being considered.

Phase II

These trials start when patients rather than healthy subjects are tested for the first time. Elimination of the drug from the body should be assessed in patients, since they may metabolize the drug differently. Phase II is usually divided into two sections: early and late. The early Phase II trials involve the administration of the drug to the patients with observations of potential therapeutic benefit and side effects. An attempt is made to establish a dose range for more definitive therapeutic trials. Late Phase II trials are intended to establish whether the new drug is efficacious in reducing the manifestations of the disease of interest and to compare its efficacy and side effects to other marketed drugs used for similar purposes.

To optimize the probability of detecting drugs that can decrease alcohol consumption, the most powerful design involves intrasubject comparison such as a cross-over design (rather than the intersubject comparisons in the early Phase II studies). Therefore, the statistical significance for the differences between treatments can be computed for each individual and not merely for the groups as a whole. These designs are more sensitive than between-subject comparisons, because of smaller error variance in the cross-over situation.

A few points require special mention. Since we usually work with unmarketed drugs that are under clinical investigation for other indications, a series of precautions must be taken. For example, one criterion for eligibility has been that subjects be heavy social drinkers (i.e., subjects who drink excessively but are neither dependent on alcohol nor have psychosocial problems). In addition, females are usually excluded to avoid potential teratogenesis. These two precautions seemed valid when we began our studies. However, since retrospective analyses of our data showed that approximately 60 to 80% of the subjects who participated in our studies were in fact problem drinkers (subjects who drink excessively but also have psychosocial problems), we believe future studies should be performed in early problem drinkers instead of heavy social drinkers. Studies to determine the behavioral, pharmacokinetic, and dynamic interactions of the drugs with ethanol are usually conducted immediately before or concurrently with the alcohol consumption studies.

Phase III

It is now generally accepted that all claims of efficacy and safety of any treatment must be supported by several well-conducted double-blind, randomized, controlled trials performed in a sufficient number of patients (10). These methods attempt to ensure that data collection is unbiased and that extraneous influences are eliminated as far as possible. The controlled clinical trial is designed to compare treatments in patients, by controlling or balancing all the possibly relevant variables except the drug. None of the serotonergic drugs which have been tested thus far have reached this phase.

Early experiences with the alcohol-sensitizing drugs are illustrative of common problems that should not be ignored. Disulfiram was introduced in 1948 as a potential treatment for chronic alcoholism. The alcohol-sensitizing drugs inhibit aldehyde dehydrogenase so that when alcohol is ingested the concentration of acetaldehyde increases, precipitating an aversive reaction (47). However, it has not been confirmed that these agents deter further drinking. Between 1948 and 1980, 135 studies claiming to assess the efficacy of alcohol-sensitizing drugs were published. Of these, 93 studies involved oral disulfiram, 18 disulfiram implants, 16 metronidazole, and 8 citrated calcium carbimide. Only 11 were randomized controlled trials and many had serious methodological problems (38). Therefore, the conclusion was that there is no scientific evidence supporting the efficacy of any of the alcohol-sensitizing drugs (38,47). Future claims about the efficacy of any drug must be supported by studies with acceptable scientific standards and which have been conducted with adequate care and proficiency.

It is also important to collect accurate information about alcohol consumption and the problems (psychosocial, biomedical) related to its excessive use. Objective measurements for assessing alcohol consumption are rarely used, but without accurate assessment of both the independent (drug) and the dependent (ethanol intake) variables, unambiguous conclusions concerning drug effects are not possible (42,44). The appropriate assessment of compliance is crucial for interpreting results of drug trials. We will analyze this aspect in detail in subsequent sections.

Phase IV

Recently, the need to conduct what is called the Phase IV, or Postmarketing Surveillance, of every new drug has been emphasized. In the years immediately following marketing, widespread use may result in the discovery of rare side effects, previously unknown drug interactions, potential new therapeutic uses, or more appropriate dosage recommendations. The recent experience that led to the withdrawal of zimelidine from the market illustrates the importance of close postmarketing monitoring of new drugs (44).

ASSESSMENT OF COMPLIANCE IN DRUG TRIALS WITH ALCOHOL ABUSERS

The assessment of compliance is essential to permit a more accurate evaluation of efficacy and safety in a new drug trial. Heavy alcohol users exhibit a low level of compliance with respect to presentation for and retention in treatment (52). Because the belief that alcohol abusers are less compliant than light drinkers or abstainers with respect to the taking of medication is widespread, despite the lack of supportive evidence, they are often excluded from clinical trials. However, they are still likely to be subjects in clinical studies involving a wide range of drugs.

Recently, we used a comprehensive strategy for assessing compliance with drug treatment and the accuracy of reported ethanol use in alcohol abusers participating in a randomized, double-blind, cross-over study testing the effect of zimelidine on ethanol consumption (42).

Identical zimelidine and placebo capsules containing a riboflavin (20 mg) marker were dispensed biweekly. A summary of the procedures used for assessing compliance is presented in Table 1. Subjects were asked to take their medication at 8 p.m., to provide urine samples 2 to 4 hr thereafter (peak of riboflavin concentration in urine) and to record daily the exact times they took the drug and collected urine. Subjects were also asked to refrain from taking vitamin preparations containing riboflavin and to inform investigators of any other medications consumed. At the end of each day they recorded the total number of standard drinks consumed (55). At biweekly assessments, their records of alcohol consumption, drug administration, and urine collection were reviewed for com-

TABLE 1. *Compliance measures*

Medication
    Riboflavin estimate[a]
    Pill count[b]
    Patient self-report[b]
    Drug and metabolite in urine[a]
    Drug and metabolite in serum[b]
    5-HT uptake inhibition[b]
Alcohol use
    Diary (number of drinks)[a]
    Urine alcohol concentration[a]
Adherence to other instructions
    Urines sent (% returned)[a]
    Appointments kept[b]

[a] daily
[b] biweekly

pleteness. The number of hours since they had ingested their last medication was recorded. They, then, underwent physical examination and screening of urine for drugs. A 60-ml blood sample was drawn for laboratory tests (hematologic, liver, and renal function) and for measuring zimelidine and norzimelidine concentrations in serum (63). Zimelidine and norzimelidine concentrations were also determined in daily urine samples. To confirm zimelidine effect on 5-HT uptake, the ability of patient's serum samples to inhibit 5-HT uptake by rat hypothalamic synaptosomes was assessed (20). Containers were returned, and the remaining capsules counted. A new prescription for the medication for the next 2 weeks was dispensed.

Compliance estimates were calculated in the following manners for the tracer (riboflavin) technique, capsule count, and self-report. For the tracer technique, a urine was judged positive if the riboflavin concentration as examined by spectrofluorescence was $> \bar{x} + 2$ SD (where $\bar{x}$ and SD are the mean and standard deviation of riboflavin concentration in urine samples in the baseline period for a given subject). Compliance was estimated as the number of positive urines per number of days in trial, expressed as a percentage. Since subjects returned unused capsules every 2 weeks, the compliance estimate for the capsule count method was calculated as the ratio of the number of capsules prescribed minus the number returned, to the number of capsules prescribed and expressed as a percentage. The compliance estimate for the self-report method was calculated as the ratio of the reported number of capsules consumed to the number of capsules prescribed and expressed as a percentage. Self-reports of alcohol consumption were recorded as the total number of drinks consumed each day, and this was correlated with the daily urine alcohol concentrations, as measured by an enzymatic assay (19).

Of the 16 subjects, 3 (Nos. 1004, 1028, and 1037) developed symptoms of drug-induced hepatitis, which led to discontinuation of zimelidine during the first dosing period (44,53), 2 subjects (Nos. 1025 and 1026) dropped out during the second zimelidine period for personal reasons, and a sixth (No. 1001) did not keep his records of alcohol consumption adequately during the last two experimental periods (42). Compliance results are presented for all subjects (Table 2). Subjects kept 100% of their appointments, and 94% of all urines were mailed in for analysis.

Each subject in the trial provided his own baseline riboflavin concentrations. The mean riboflavin concentration in urine showed a 5- to 6-fold increase on the average (42). The overall minimum mean compliance estimate according to this procedure was 78%. Individual compliance ratings are recorded in Table 2. At least one subject (No. 1028) was unable to comply with the advice of not taking vitamin supplements containing riboflavin, and, thus, his data are unreliable in terms of determining compliance based on riboflavin data.

Table 2 also shows individual and mean zimelidine and norzimelidine concentrations in serum and urine and reductions in serotonin uptake during the zimelidine periods. All these measurements indicated a high level of compliance. No significant serum drug concentrations were detected in the placebo periods, confirming that there were no prescribing errors. Low concentrations of zimelidine and more particularly norzimelidine were detected in the first few days of the placebo period when it followed a drug period.

Capsule count indicated a mean compliance estimate of 97% (with a range of 89% to 100%) for the duration of the time spent in the trial (Table 2). Self-report of medications consumed also showed high compliance. The mean result was 97% (range 88 to 100%). Two subjects did not record this information (Table 2).

The number of daily drinks reported by the subjects correlated with the alcohol concentrations in the urine ($r = 0.62$, $p < 0.001$). The individual correlations ranged from 0.45 to 0.73 (Table 2). Therefore, daily urine ethanol concentrations correlated well with self-report, and urine ethanol concentrations were highest when collection of urine samples coincided with the time of maximum alcohol consumption.

This study illustrates a high degree of compliance in a group of alcohol abusers participating in a trial with a new drug. These results have implications for trial design and for the assessment of efficacy and toxicity of drugs in these subjects.

It is essential that a high degree of compliance be attained in a given trial in order that a confident assessment of the efficacy of the drug be made. Changes in relevant dependent variables in clinical trials (in this case, variation in ethanol intake) are often dependent on a variety of nonpharmacological factors. Therefore, it is important to determine that the subjects have taken the agent in order to attribute a change to a genuine drug effect. Since our subjects were highly compliant, we can more confidently state that variations in alcohol intake were induced by zimelidine. Accurate assessment of compliance in clinical trials also facilitates the detection and assessment of drug-induced toxicity. Establishing a causal relationship between adverse effects and drug administration is difficult, because manifestations of adverse drug reactions are usually not unique (37). In

TABLE 2. Subject compliance characteristics

Subject no.	Age (years)	Days in trial	Urines returned (%)	Appointments kept (%)	Compliance estimate (%)			Urine/ ethanol correlations (r)	Percentage decrease in 5-HT uptake during zimelidine treatment relative to baseline	Mean drug concentrations in body fluids during zimelidine treatment			
					Riboflavin	Pill count	Self-report			Blood (ng/ml)		Urine (μg/ml)	
										Z	NZ	Z	NZ
1001[c]	34	28	100	100	39	100	[a]	0.73	67.1	25.4	124.1	0.52	4.66
1004[d]	49	26	100	100	69	100	[a]	0.45	[a]	102.2	103.2	1.57	5.00
1006	29	56	100	100	91	96	96	0.58	79.9	22.5	63.7	7.95	16.69
1007	33	56	100	100	79	100	100	0.58	78.0	31.0	110.0	3.46	9.89
1008	22	56	95	100	94	100	98	0.68	47.6	43.5	132.5	2.38	8.21
1011	24	56	100	100	88	96	98	0.59	41.6	27.4	100.4	1.19	3.82
1013	24	56	98	100	91	100	10	0.70	43.4	20.9	109.6	1.73	5.98
1023	45	56	98	100	85	96	96	0.54	47.6	52.1	122.8	1.23	5.65
1024	51	56	93	100	91	95	98	0.60	46.6	33.9	101.4	16.54	18.39
1025[e]	36	50	96	100	85	100	100	0.59	38.7	43.3	135.2	3.02	8.76
1026[e]	42	44	84	100	78	89	88	0.67	58.5	22.3	103.6	3.00	8.38
1027	46	56	100	100	88	98	100	0.56	50.7	84.8	135.2	4.70	10.64
1028[d]	32	27	96	100	[b]	96	100	0.38	[a]	[a]	[a]	6.13	5.17
1034	26	56	98	100	98	100	100	0.63	49.3	48.3	116.7	3.03	6.27
1036	34	56	86	100	63	95	95	0.64	50.9	67.8	138.7	2.01	3.06
1037[d]	33	21	62	100	38	100	92	0.63	[a]	72.6	102.5	5.81	5.49
Group means	35	47	94	100	78	98	97	0.62	53.82	46.5	113.3	4.02	7.88

[a] No data available.
[b] Subject ingested vitamins containing riboflavin.
[c] Subject did not adhere to protocol during placebo 2 and drug 2 periods (data are excluded from these periods).
[d] Treatment discontinued because of suspected adverse drug reaction.
[e] Subjects dropped out during second drug period for personal reasons.
Z, zimelidine; NZ, norzimelidine.

addition, subjects are usually receiving several medications. The conclusive demonstration of the presence of zimelidine and norzimelidine, while three subjects presented with significant alterations in liver enzymes, permitted a more precise assessment of the contribution of zimelidine to the toxic effects (44,54).

Direct measurement of the drug and metabolite in the blood and urine and the measurement of uptake of serotonin confirmed that all subjects were taking drug in the drug periods and no drug in the placebo periods. Similarly, both indirect methods, capsule count and self-reporting, indicated an exceptionally high rate of compliance. The average compliance estimate was 97% with both methods compared to 78% with the riboflavin technique. Studies in clinical practice have also demonstrated a tendency for the pill count technique to possibly overestimate compliance (3,51). There is limited but similar evidence from other clinical trials that direct methods determine lower levels of compliance than indirect methods (26).

In summary then, we demonstrated that high compliance can exist in a group of heavy alcohol users when stringent selection procedures and multiple ways to measure and possibly reinforce compliance are used. From a practical viewpoint, we would suggest a minimum requirement of a combination of one objective measure (direct method) together with one or more indirect methods for all drug trials. This would enable investigators to make confident statements about drug efficacy and toxicity. These assessments of compliance are particularly important for validating results when trials are conducted in subjects reputed to exhibit poor compliance (e.g., alcohol abusers).

STUDIES WITH SEROTONERGIC DRUGS

Central 5-HT Function and Ethanol Intake

Our search for new drugs has focused on agents that enhance central serotonergic function, because they consistently attenuate ethanol consumption. The clinical importance of 5-HT and 5-HT-altering drugs became apparent by the recent demonstration that the 5-HT uptake inhibitors zimelidine (1,42) and citalopram (41) attenuate ethanol intake in humans. Such findings suggest an innovative approach for pharmacologically moderating alcohol consumption.

Effects of Serotonergic Drugs on Ethanol Intake in Experimental Animals

Animal studies have shown that pharmacological manipulations of central 5-HT (5-hydroxytryptamine) neurotransmission alter ethanol consumption and preference. The more consistent findings have been obtained with direct and indirect 5-HT agonists. Ethanol intake decreases after the administration of (a) 5-HT precursors such as tryptophan (65) and 5-hydroxytryptophan

(11,34,62,64,65), (b) intracerebral 5-HT (13), and (c) postsynaptic 5-HT agonists such as MK-212 (22) and quipazine (64). However, increases in ethanol intake have been reported in a few studies in which tryptophan was administered in the diet (32,59). All 5-HT uptake inhibitors tested including zimelidine (21,50), norzimelidine (49), citalopram (41,49), alaproclate (49), fluoxetine (64), fluvoxamine (22), indalpine (23), and viqualine (41), consistently and repeatedly have been shown to diminish ethanol intake when offered as a free-choice with water. The effect of 5-HT uptake inhibitors on ethanol intake has also been tested in genetically inbred animals that are ethanol-preferring. For example, fluoxetine decreased ethanol intake in P rats (28) and zimelidine, citalopram, and fluvoxamine reduced ethanol intake and preference in UChB rats. (J. Mardones et al., 1985, *personal communication*). Since zimelidine did not alter ethanol consumption in C57BL-6J mice, this effect may be species-specific (41). Moreover, it has been shown that monoamine uptake inhibitors, which do not inhibit 5-HT uptake specifically, do not alter ethanol intake (49). For instance, amitriptyline [which moderately inhibits both 5-HT and norepinephrine (NE) uptake], desmethylimipramine, and doxepin (both selective inhibitors of NE uptake) did not have an effect on ethanol intake (49).

If 5-HT plays an important role in regulating ethanol intake, then decreases in 5-HT function in the CNS would be expected to result in increased ethanol intake. The destruction of 5-HT-containing neurons with the neurotoxins 5,6- or 5,7-dihydroxytryptamine (5,6- or 5,7-DHT) has been usually reported to enhance ethanol intake (15,27,31,48). However, studies with parachlorophenylalanine (PCPA), which inhibits 5-HT synthesis, have given conflicting results. Ethanol intake has been reported to be increased (11), decreased (5,9,33,45,60–62), or unaltered (5,14,16,46) after PCPA treatment. These discrepancies may be explained by the lack of comparable laboratory conditions and/or methodological problems. For example, in most of the studies, PCPA was administered orally, possibly resulting in erratic drug absorption and gastrointestinal side effects. Postsynaptic receptor antagonists have been reported to increase (12) or have no effect on ethanol intake (2).

Effects of 5-HT Uptake Inhibitors on Ethanol Intake in Humans

The 5-HT uptake inhibitors zimelidine (1,42) and citalopram (43) have been tested in alcohol abusers. These studies have demonstrated that these drugs do attenuate ethanol intake in alcohol abusers, providing strong support for a role of 5-HT in regulating ethanol intake in humans and cross-validating the results obtained in experimental animals. Consequently, the simple free-choice paradigm is a valid test for screening new pharmacological interventions.

We tested the effect of zimelidine (200 mg p.o.) on ethanol intake in 16 non-depressed, healthy, heavy drinkers (≥4 drinks/day) in a double-blind, randomized, double cross-over trial (42). Zimelidine decreased the number of drinks consumed and increased the percentage of days of abstinence. Since subjects were not clinically depressed, and zimelidine's effect on alcohol intake occurred in less than 2 weeks, such variations could not have been due to its antidepressant action. Marked interindividual variations in the pattern of response to zimelidine were observed. Approximately 50% of subjects were responders, 35% partial responders, and 15% nonresponders (41,42).

In another recently completed double-blind, randomized, cross-over trial, we studied the effect of citalopram (20 mg/day p.o. or 40 mg/day p.o.), the most specific and selective 5-HT uptake inhibitor (17), on ethanol intake in nondepressed, healthy heavy drinkers. Citalopram (40 mg/day p.o.) significantly decreased the number of drinks consumed and increased the number of days of abstinence (43).

CONCLUSIONS

The identification and testing of new drugs to decrease alcohol consumption provide many challenges to basic and clinical investigators. The experience of the past years emphasize the importance of the following:

1. Studies to identify the psychobiologic mechanisms of excessive alcohol consumption could lead to more effective drug therapies.

2. The systematic testing for drugs that could decrease alcohol consumption should be undertaken by some pharmaceutical companies.

3. The quality of clinical studies for currently available drugs could be improved by the use of acceptable scientific standards to test efficacy and toxicity. Most of the methodology to accomplish this is available.

4. 5-HT agonists, particularly 5-HT uptake inhibitors, consistently moderate ethanol intake in experimental animals and humans. The results with zimelidine and citalopram provide strong support to the hypothesis that 5-HT plays a role in regulating ethanol intake in humans. These drugs may provide an innovative approach for moderating ethanol intake in problem drinkers. Clinical studies for testing their potential as treatments should be undertaken.

ACKNOWLEDGMENTS

We gratefully acknowledge the help of Dr. V. Khouw, Dr. S. L. Lee, Ms. D. Woodley, Ms. K. Kadlec, Ms. M. Harrison, Ms. K. Kaplan, and Ms. K. Sykora for the conduct of the human studies. We also thank Ms. C. Van Der Giessen for typing the manuscript and Ms. K. Kadlec for her careful editing of the manuscript.

These studies have been supported by the Intramural Grant Program of the Addiction Research Foundation of Ontario.

REFERENCES

1. Amit, Z., Brown, Z., Sutherland, A., Rockman, G., Gill, K., and Selvaggi, N. (1985): Reduction in alcohol intake in humans as a function of treatment with zimelidine: Implications for treatment. In: *Research Advances in New Psychopharmacological Treatments for Alcoholism,* edited by C. A. Naranjo and E. M. Sellers, pp. 189–198. Elsevier Science Publishers B. V., Amsterdam.
2. Amit, Z., Sutherland, E. A., Gill, K., and Ogren, S. O. (1984): Zimelidine: A review of its effects on ethanol consumption. *Neurosci. Biobehav. Rev.,* 8:35–54.
3. Bergman, A. B., and Werner, R. J. (1963): Failure of children to receive penicillin by mouth. *N. Engl. J. Med.,* 268:1334–1338.
4. Cicero, T. J. (1980): Animal models of alcoholism and alcohol drinking. In: *Animal Models in Alcohol Research,* edited by K. Eriksson, J. D. Sinclair, and K. Kiianmaa, pp. 99–117. Academic Press, New York.
5. Cicero, T. J., and Hill, S. Y. (1970): Ethanol self-selection in rats: A distinction between absolute and 95% ethanol. *Physiol. Behav.,* 5:787–791.
6. Deitrich, R. A., and Melchior, C. L. (1985): A critical assessment of animal models for testing new drugs for altering ethanol intake. In: *Research Advances in New Psychopharmacological Treatments for Alcoholism,* edited by C. A. Naranjo and E. M. Sellers, pp. 23–41. Elsevier Science Publishers B. V., Amsterdam.
7. Edwards, G. (1984): Drug treatments for drinking problems: Finding a way forward. In: *Pharmacological Treatments for Alcoholism,* edited by G. Edwards and J. Littleton, pp. 3–11. Methuen Inc., New York.
8. Edwards, G., and Littleton, J., editors (1984): *Pharmacological Treatments for Alcoholism.* Methuen Inc., New York.
9. Frey, H.-H., Magnussen, M. P., and Kaergaard-Nielsen, C. (1970): The effect of p-chloroamphetamine on the consumption of ethanol by rats. *Arch. Int. Pharmacodyn. Ther.,* 183:165–172.
10. Friedman, L. M., Furberg, C. D., and de Mets, D. C., editors (1985): *Fundamentals of Clinical Trials, Second Edition.* John Wright PSG Inc., Boston.
11. Geller, I. (1973): Effects of para-chlorophenyl alanine and 5-hydroxytryptophan on alcohol intake in the rat. *Pharmacol. Biochem. Behav.,* 1:361–365.
12. Geller, I., Hartmann, R. J., and Messiha, F. S. (1975): Effects of cinanserin, a serotonin antagonist on ethanol preference in the rat. *Proc. West. Pharmacol. Soc.,* 18:141–145.
13. Hill, S. Y. (1974): Intraventricular injection of 5-hydroxytryptamine and alcohol consumption in rats. *Biol. Psychiatry,* 8:151–158.
14. Hill, S. Y., and Goldstein, R. (1974): Effect of p-chlorophenylalanine and stress on alcohol consumption by rats. *Quart. J. Studies Alcohol,* 35:34–41.
15. Ho, A. K. S., Tsai, C. S., Chen, R. C. A., Begleiter, H., and Kissin, B. (1974): Experimental studies on alcoholism: I. Increase in alcohol preference by 5,6-dihydroxytryptamine and brain acetylcholine. *Psychopharmacologia,* 40:101–107.
16. Holman, R. B., Hoyland, V., and Shillito, E. E. (1975): The failure of p-chlorophenylalanine to affect voluntary alcohol consumption in rats. *Br. J. Pharmacol.,* 53:299–304.
17. Hyttel, J., and Larsen, J.-J. (1985): Neuropharmacological mechanisms of serotonin re-uptake inhibitors. In: *Research Advances in New Psychopharmacological Treatments for Alcoholism,* edited by C. A. Naranjo and E. M. Sellers, pp. 107–119. Elsevier Science Publishers B. V., Amsterdam.
18. Kalant, H. (1985): Interactions of ethanol and neuropeptides. In: *Research Advances in New Psychopharmacological Treatments for Alcoholism,* edited by C. A. Naranjo and E. M. Sellers, pp. 69–82. Elsevier Science Publishers B. V., Amsterdam.
19. Kapur, B., and Anderson, M. (1980): Enzymatic determination of ethanol in urine with the American Monitor KDA. *Clin. Chem.,* 26:1063.
20. Koide, T., and Uyemura, K. (1980): A comparison of the inhibitory effects of new non-tricyclic amine uptake inhibitors on the uptake of norepinephrine and 5-hydroxytryptamine into synaptosomes of the rat brain. *Neuropharmacology,* 19:349–354.
21. Lawrin, M., Naranjo, C. A., and Sellers, E. M. (1983): Studies on the mechanism of zimelidine-induced decrease in alcohol consumption in rats. *Proc. Can. Fed. Biol. Soc.,* 26:116.
22. Lawrin, M. O., Naranjo, C. A., and Sellers, E. M. (1985): Enhanced serotonergic neurotransmission decreases ethanol consumption. Consistent results with a serotonin agonist. *Proc. Can. Fed. Biol. Soc.,* 28:81.

23. Le Bourhis, B., Uzan, A., Aufrere, G., and Le Fur, G. (1981): Effets de l'indalpine, inhibiteur spécifique de la recapture de la serotonine sur la dependance comportementale a l'ethanol et sur la prise volontaire d'alcool chez le rat. *Ann. Pharm. Fr.,* 39:11–20.
24. Lester, D., and Freed, E. X. (1973): Criteria for an animal model of alcoholism. *Pharmacol. Biochem. Behav.,* 1:103–107.
25. Mardones, J., Segovia-Riquelme, N., and Contreras, S. (1984): Effects of sulpiride on the voluntary consumption of ethanol, water and solid food by UChA and UChB rats. *IRCS Med. Sci.,* 12: 600–601.
26. Mattson, M. E. (1982): Compliance patterns in AMIS. *Controlled Clin. Trials,* 3:137.
27. Melchoir, C. L., and Myers, R. D. (1976): Genetic difference in ethanol drinking of the rat following injection of 5-OHDA, 5,6-DHT or 5,7-DHT into the cerebral ventricles. *Pharmacol. Biochem. Behav.,* 5:63–72.
28. Murphy, J. M., Waller, M. B., Gatto, G. J., McBride, W. J., Lumeng, L., and Li, T. K. (1985): Monoamine uptake inhibitors attenuate ethanol intake in alcohol-preferring (P) rats. *Alcohol,* 2(2):349–352.
29. Murray, R. M. (1980): Why are the drug companies so disinterested in alcoholism? *Br. J. Addict.,* 75:113–115.
30. Myers, R. D., and Ewing, J. A. (1980): Aversive factors in alcohol drinking in humans and animals. *Pharmacol. Biochem. Behav.,* 13(Suppl. 1):269–277.
31. Myers, R. D., and Melchior, C. L. (1975): Alcohol drinking in the rat after destruction of serotonergic and catecholaminergic neurons in the brain. *Res. Commun. Chem. Pathol. Pharmacol.,* 19:363–378.
32. Myers, R. D., and Melchior, C. L. (1975): Dietary tryptophan and the selection of ethyl alcohol in different strains of rats. *Psychopharmacologia,* 42:109–115.
33. Myers, R. D., and Veale, W. L. (1968): Alcohol preference in the rat: Reduction following depletion of brain serotonin. *Science,* 160:1469–1471.
34. Myers, R. D., and Veale, W. L. (1972): The determinants of alcohol preference in animals. In: *Biology of Alcoholism, Volume II,* edited by H. Begleiter and B. Kissin, pp. 131–168. Plenum Press, New York.
35. Naranjo, C. A. (1983): Recent advances in the pharmacotherapy of alcoholism. In: *Clinical Pharmacology and Therapeutics,* edited by M. Velasco, pp. 132–139. Excerpta Medica, Amsterdam.
36. Naranjo, C. A. (1985): Drug treatments for alcoholism: The need for innovation. In: *Research Advances in New Psychopharmacological Treatments for Alcoholism,* edited by C. A. Naranjo and E. M. Sellers, pp. 1–9. Elsevier Science Publishers B. V., Amsterdam.
37. Naranjo, C. A., Busto, U., Sellers, E. M., Sandor, P., Ruiz, I., Roberts, E. A., Janecek, E., Domecq, C., and Greenblatt, D. J. (1981): A method for estimating the probability of adverse drug reactions. *Clin. Pharmacol. Ther.,* 30:239–245.
38. Naranjo, C. A., Cappell, H., and Sellers, E. M. (1981): Pharmacological control of alcohol consumption: Tactics for the identification and testing of new drugs. *Addict. Behav.,* 6:261–269.
39. Naranjo, C. A., and Janecek, E. (1985): Drug development and regulations. In: *Principles of Medical Pharmacology, Fourth Edition,* edited by H. Kalant, W. H. E. Roschlau, and E. M. Sellers, pp. 837–847. University of Toronto Press, Toronto.
40. Naranjo, C. A., and Sellers, E. M., editors (1985): *Research Advances in New Psychopharmacological Treatments for Alcoholism.* Elsevier Science Publishers B. V., Amsterdam.
41. Naranjo, C. A., Sellers, E. M., and Lawrin, M. O. (1986): Modulation of ethanol intake by serotonin uptake inhibitors. *J. Clin. Psychiatry,* 47(4):16–22.
42. Naranjo, C. A., Sellers, E. M., Roach, C. A., Woodley, D. V., Sanchez-Craig, M., and Sykora, K. (1984): Zimelidine-induced variations in alcohol intake by nondepressed heavy drinkers. *Clin. Pharmacol. Ther.,* 35:374–381.
43. Naranjo, C. A., Sellers, E. M., Sullivan, J. T., Woodley, D. V., Kadlec, K., and Sykora, K. (1986): Serotonin uptake inhibitors (SUI) consistently moderate ethanol intake (EI) in humans: Citalopram (C) effects. *Clin. Pharmacol. Ther.,* 39(2):215.
44. Naranjo, C. A., Sellers, E. M., Wu, P. H., and Lawrin, M. (1985): Moderation of ethanol intake: Role of enhanced serotonergic neurotransmission. In: *Research Advances in New Psychopharmacological Treatments for Alcoholism,* edited by C. A. Naranjo and E. M. Sellers, pp. 171–186. Elsevier Science Publishers B. V., Amsterdam.
45. Opitz, K. (1969): Beobachtungen bei alkohol trinkenden ratten—einfluss von fenfluramin. *Pharmakopsychiatr. Neuro-Psychopharmakol.,* 2:202–205.

46. Parker, L. F., and Radow, B. L. (1976): Effects of parachlorophenylalanine on ethanol self-selection in the rat. *Pharmacol. Biochem. Behav.,* 4:535–540.
47. Peachey, J. E., and Naranjo, C. A. (1983): The use of disulfiram and other alcohol-sensitizing drugs in the treatment of alcoholism. In: *Research Advances in Alcohol and Drug Problems, Volume 7,* edited by Y. Israel, F. G. Glaser, H. Kalant, R. E. Popham, W. Schmidt, and R. E. Smart, pp. 397–431. Plenum Publishing Corporation, New York.
48. Richardson, J. S., and Novakovski, D. M. (1978): Brain monoamines and free choice ethanol consumption in rats. *Drug Alcohol Depend.,* 3:253–264.
49. Rockman, G. E., Amit, Z., Brown, Z. W., Bourque, C., and Ogren, S. O. (1982): An investigation of the mechanisms of action of 5-hydroxytryptamine in the suppression of ethanol intake. *Neuropharmacology,* 21:341–347.
50. Rockman, G. E., Amit, Z., Carr, G., Brown, Z. W., and Ogren, S. O. (1979): Attenuation of ethanol intake by 5-hydroxytryptamine uptake blockade in laboratory rats. I. Involvement of brain 5-hydroxytryptamine in the mediation of the positive reinforcing of ethanol. *Arch. Int. Pharmacodyn. Ther.,* 241:245–259.
51. Roth, H. P., Caron, H. S., and Hsi, B. P. (1970): Measuring intake of a prescribed medication. A bottle count and a tracer technique compared. *Clin. Pharmacol. Ther.,* 11:228–237.
52. Sellers, E. M., Cappell, H. D., and Marshman, J. A. (1979): Compliance in the control of alcohol abuse. In: *Compliance in Health Care,* edited by R. B. Haynes, D. W. Taylor, and D. L. Sackett, pp. 223–243. The Johns Hopkins University Press, Baltimore.
53. Sellers, E. M., Naranjo, C. A., and Peachey, J. E. (1981): Drugs to decrease alcohol consumption. *N. Engl. J. Med.,* 305:1255–1262.
54. Sellers, E. M., Vidins, E. A., Engels, F., Fan, T., and Naranjo, C. A. (1983): Clinical and experimental studies on zimelidine-induced hepatoxicity. In: *Proc. II World Conf. Clin. Pharmacol. Ther.,* p. 93.
55. Skinner, H. A. (1984): Assessing alcohol use by patients in treatment. In: *Research Advances in Alcohol and Drug Problems, Volume 8,* edited by R. G. Smart, H. D. Cappell, F. B. Glaser, Y. Israel, H. Kalant, R. E. Popham, W. Schmidt, and E. M. Sellers, pp. 183–207. Plenum Press, New York.
56. Skinner, H. A. (1985): The clinical spectrum of alcoholism: Implications for new drug therapies. In: *Research Advances in New Psychopharmacological Treatments for Alcoholism,* edited by C. A. Naranjo and E. M. Sellers, pp. 123–135. Elsevier Science Publishers B. V., Amsterdam.
57. Skinner, H. A., and Holt, S. (1983): Early intervention for alcohol problems. *J. R. Coll. Gen. Pract.,* 33:787–791.
58. Smith, B. R., Amit, Z., Aragon, C. M. G., and Socaransky, S. M. (1985): Neurobiological correlates of ethanol self-administration: The role of acetaldehyde. In: *Research Advances in New Psychopharmacological Treatments for Alcoholism,* edited by C. A. Naranjo and E. M. Sellers, pp. 45–63. Elsevier Science Publishers B. V., Amsterdam.
59. Sprince, H., Parker, C. M., Smith, G. G., and Gonzales, L. J. (1972): Alcoholism: Biochemical and nutritional aspects of brain amines, aldehydes and amino acids. *Nutr. Rep. Int.,* 5:185–200.
60. Stein, J. M., Wayner, M. J., and Tilson, H. A. (1977): The effect of parachlorophenylalanine on the intake of ethanol and saccharin solutions. *Pharmacol. Biochem. Behav.,* 6:117–122.
61. Veale, W. L., and Myers, R. D. (1970): Decrease in ethanol intake in the rats following administration of p-chlorophenylalanine. *Neuropharmacology,* 9:317–326.
62. Walters, J. K. (1977): Effects of PCPA on the consumption of alcohol, water and other solutions. *Pharmacol. Biochem. Behav.,* 6:377–383.
63. Westerlund, D., and Erikson, E. (1979): Reversed-phase chromatography of zimelidine and similar dibasic amines. 1. Analysis in biological material. *J. Chromatogr.,* 185:593–603.
64. Zabik, J. E., Binkerd, K., and Roache, J. D. (1985): Serotonin and ethanol aversion in the rat. In: *Research Advances in New Psychopharmacological Treatments for Alcoholism,* edited by C. A. Naranjo and E. M. Sellers, pp. 87–101. Elsevier Science Publishers B. V., Amsterdam.
65. Zabik, J. E., Liao, S.-S., Jeffreys, M., and Maickel, R. P. (1978): The effects of DL-5-hydroxytryptophan on ethanol consumption by rats. *Res. Commun. Chem. Pathol. Pharmacol.,* 20:69–78.

Brain Reward Systems and Abuse, edited by
J. Engel and L. Oreland.
Raven Press, New York © 1987.

Nicotine Reward: Studies of Abuse Liability and Physical Dependence Potential

*Jack E. Henningfield, *Edythe D. London,
and *Jerome H. Jaffe

*National Institute on Drug Abuse Addiction Research Center,
Baltimore, Maryland 21224

In theory at least, a drug that produces reward may reinforce the behavior which leads to its administration. Such a drug may be abused when made available to a susceptible population. Nonetheless, a drug which does not produce reward might still be a reinforcer (e.g., if it alleviates some aversive state). Whether such drugs have a high potential for abuse is not well established. The ability of rewarding drugs to act as reinforcers is linked conceptually but complexly to the notion of drug abuse (cf. refs. 4 and 37). Thus, most drugs that are abused also serve as reinforcers, and many of these drugs also produce physical (physiologic) dependence.

Laboratory studies use a variety of techniques to assess drug effects and to estimate the likelihood that a drug will be abused, produce physical dependence, and lead to the complex behavior we designate as drug dependence or addiction. These techniques include self-administration paradigms, place-preference tests, assessment of the degree to which the stimulus properties of the drug generalize to the stimulus properties of known drugs of abuse, and measures of tolerance and physical dependence produced by repeated drug administration. Adjunctive assessments include measurements of effects considered beneficial to the individual such as performance enhancement and weight reduction. Most of these techniques are used with either animal or human subjects.

These laboratory procedures are ways to gauge some element of the behavior that constitutes drug dependence. As predictors, the validity and reliability of each procedure is imperfect. For example, they provide little information about nonpharmacologic factors that influence the actual incidence of drug abuse and drug dependence. Such nonpharmacological factors are numerous and include the price and availability of the drug, the social status conferred by use of the drug, and genetic predisposition to be reinforced by a specific drug. Despite these limitations, laboratory studies can provide a basis for predicting the likelihood that use of a substance may cause drug dependence and for understanding the mechanisms that underlie that process.

For the sake of clarity, several key words are defined below as they are used in this chapter. The term "drug dependence" is used in accord with the suggestions of a recent World Health Organization memorandum, which describes drug dependence as a complex behavioral pattern in which the use of a drug takes priority over other values in life (61). Drug dependence, which is not an all-or-none phenomenon, is also defined by its relationship to the pharmacological activity of the substance. In this regard, it is substance-seeking behavior that is determined by the CNS activity of a constituent drug. Tolerance and physical dependence (withdrawal phenomenon) may or may not be present. The term "addiction" has been used so generally and variably that it has lost much of its technical usefulness and is not used in the remainder of this chapter. Evaluation of the potential of a substance to produce drug dependence includes the testing of its "abuse liability" and "physical dependence potential" (4,37). "Abuse liability" refers to those effects of a drug that result in its self-administration, often in the face of mounting cost, physical and social dysfunction, and to the sacrifice of more socially-acceptable behavior (see also ref. 36). "Physical dependence potential" refers to the direct physiological effects produced by repeated administration of the drug, such that neuroadaptation ("physiologic" or "physical dependence") occurs (see also ref. 32). Neuroadaptation is assessed by the demonstration of tolerance to the drug's effects and physiologic rebound phenomena ("abstinence" or "withdrawal") following termination of drug administration or the administration of an antagonist. Neuroadaptation is a frequent but not invariant correlate of abuse liability; however, it may interact with abuse liability, and it often is relevant in the treatment of drug dependence. An additional concept central to many discussions of drug dependence is the damage or debilitation produced by the drug. It is well known that such damage may occur over the long-term with tobacco use (cf. ref. 54).

Tobacco is commonly used in a variety of ways, including deep inhalation of cigarette smoke, inhalation of pipe and cigar smoke, and consumption of smokeless forms of tobacco including snuff and chewing tobacco. A prescription form of nicotine in the form of a chewing gum (polacrilex) also is available for treatment of tobacco dependence. Centuries of historical observation, anecdotal insight, and scientific research have suggested that nicotine produces many of the effects that result in compulsive tobacco use (8,22). The evidence includes similarities between the compulsive use of tobacco and that of drugs such as opioids, stimulants, and alcohol. Studies of the pharmacokinetics and distribution of nicotine are consistent with the hypothesis that tobacco self-administration is a form of drug dependence. However, such observations provide only indirect evidence concerning the abuse liability and dependence potential of nicotine itself. Obtaining direct evidence that tobacco use is primarily the self-administration of nicotine and not merely a habitual behavior such as jogging or television watching is not just semantic; the implications are fundamental to issues of public health, legislative jurisdiction, and treatment of the behavior.

The literature relevant to the abuse liability and dependence potential of tobacco may be divided into two general categories. The first is a systematic comparison of tobacco with prototypic dependence-producing substances. Such a comparison shows that patterns of use and effects of tobacco share critical points of commonality with the consumption of alcoholic beverages, opium, coca leaf, and cannabis. The similarities distinguish tobacco (the substance) from other substances such as food, and tobacco use (the behavior) from habitual behaviors such as television watching and exercise, which are not associated with the ingestion of a substance. The second body of relevant data concerns direct evaluations of the abuse liability and dependence potential of nicotine itself. These data confirm the fact that nicotine meets rigorous experimental criteria as a drug that has a liability for abuse and the potential to produce physical dependence. Thus, it appears that the abuse potential of tobacco depends on its ability to serve as a source of nicotine.

RELATION OF TOBACCO USE TO DRUG DEPENDENCE

The basis for the categorization of tobacco as a dependence-producing substance and for compulsive tobacco self-administration as a form of drug dependence is that, when systematically compared to prototypic drugs of abuse, tobacco (nicotine) is similar along most points of comparison. Table 1 summarizes some of these similarities (for reviews see refs. 25, 33–35, 44 and 46). There are also differences between tobacco use and other forms of substance use. For example, tobacco use is legal, widely accepted, and occurs with relatively little disruption to cognitive and behavioral performance.

The similarities indicated in Table 1 do not provide all of the critical elements needed to distinguish the use of a substance as reflecting drug dependence, which is a special and distinct subset of habitual behaviors. Such a distinction requires that use of the substance delivers a specific drug to the CNS and that the drug produces behavioral and physiological effects characteristic of prototypic dependence-producing drugs. Thus, use of opium, coca derivatives, or alcoholic beverages results in the delivery of morphine, cocaine, or ethanol, respectively. The analogous substance in tobacco is nicotine.

TABLE 1. *Commonalities between tobacco use and drug dependence*

Spread like an infectious disease and is persistent
Patterns of relapse are generally similar following treatment
Use persists at expense and ultimate damage to individual and society
Personality types marked by elevated psychopathy and extroversion scores
A centrally acting (CNS) substance is delivered at effective dose levels by the commonly used
routes and forms of administration
The drug is a reinforcer for animals
Deprivation increases drug-seeking behavior
Patterns of self-administration and dose-response functions are orderly
"Beneficial effects" may be produced such as mood and performance enhancement, which
may occur either directly or as a function of neurohormone release

Another point of commonality among substances of abuse has implications for drug-induced reward. It is that tobacco, like other abused substances, produces effects, apart from euphoria, that may be considered to be of utility or benefit to the user.[1] Most abused drugs had specific therapeutic applications historically (e.g., refs. 2 and 5). Currently, although tobacco is not prescribed as a medicine, it is reported by users to have the following useful actions: appetite suppression, anxiety relief, regulation of arousal (via stimulant or relaxant effects), and modulation of mood.[2] The degree to which the occurrence of these effects of nicotine depend upon an individual's history of nicotine use or dependence remains to be thoroughly investigated. Similar issues remain unresolved for other drugs of abuse. The enhancement of learning and cognitive performance by nicotine has been reviewed elsewhere (58–60). Although the euphoriant properties of drugs can stand apart from collateral beneficial actions (as is also the case with morphine, amphetamine, and alcohol), attention to these other drug effects may enhance the understanding of the mechanisms underlying the dependence process.

Since nicotine, in the form of tobacco, is relatively inexpensive and widely available in a convenient form for precise dose regulation, it can provide an ideal means of self-medication of the cigarette smoker. These conditions, as well as the fact that the use of tobacco is relatively well tolerated by society may contribute to the abuse liability of tobacco. Furthermore, nicotine's brief effects, which result in frequent and repetitive behavior, ensure many opportunities to link nicotine's effects with environmental circumstances (i.e., conditioning).

A qualitative comparison of the effects produced by tobacco and other substances of abuse and the patterns of behavior that such substances engender (Table 1) provides evidence that tobacco use is an orderly form of behavior, reflecting drug dependence. Tobacco self-administration results in the delivery of a centrally active drug (nicotine), and that drug appears critical to the control of tobacco self-administration. The next section reviews recent studies in which the abuse liability and dependence potential of nicotine were directly evaluated and the role of nicotine itself specifically assessed using the same methods and procedures used to evaluate other substances of abuse.

RECENT STUDIES OF THE ABUSE LIABILITY AND DEPENDENCE POTENTIAL OF NICOTINE

If nicotine's role in the abuse liability of tobacco is like that of the psychoactive agents present in other substances of abuse (e.g., cocaine in coca leaves), then

---

[1] The term therapeutic is often used to describe such effects but may be misleading when applied to a substance that causes death and disease.

[2] It is noteworthy that all of these effects ascribed to nicotine are effects for which drugs of proven efficacy are generally available only on a prescription basis and are regulated by the U.S. Food and Drug Administration.

nicotine per se, in the absence of the multitude of stimuli associated with cigarette smoking, should meet criteria as a dependence-producing substance. Objective methods for abuse liability and physical dependence potential assessment were available before the recent interest in nicotine (4,37). These methods were adapted to studies of nicotine, with consideration given to the fact that nicotine has a more rapid onset and termination of effects than many other drugs of abuse. These methods were initially developed in studies of morphine and morphine-like drugs using human subjects (4,36,37).

The hypotheses tested are that (a) the drug in question is psychoactive, (b) it serves as a euphoriant, and (c) it acts as a reinforcer. Psychoactivity and euphoria are determined by obtaining the subject's self-reports of the drug's effects. The data are validated by behavioral and physiologic responses observed by the investigator (36). Testing whether the drug can serve as a reinforcer is accomplished by assessing the ability of the drug to strengthen and maintain orderly patterns of self-administration when the subject is permitted access to the drug (26). Physical dependence potential studies also may be conducted using previously validated procedures (e.g., refs. 37 and 43). The most commonly employed method is to assess the effects that occur when repeated drug administration is abruptly terminated (withdrawal). Another method is the substitution approach, in which the active drug is removed and replaced with either placebo or another test compound. Such studies have shown that nicotine in all commonly used forms, including the polacrilex (nicotine gum), may produce physical dependence. The polacrilex form appears to have the lowest abuse liability but is the only form available by written prescription as a controlled pharmaceutical (1). Some of the more recent findings are summarized below.

Abuse Liability Studies of Nicotine: Psychoactivity and Euphoria

In one study (28), volunteers were given nicotine and placebo under double-blind conditions. Individuals with histories of drug abuse were used as subjects because they could accurately discriminate compounds with a potential for abuse. Nicotine was given both intravenously and in the form of tobacco smoke from research cigarettes, over a range of doses, to eight subjects. The subjects inhaled smoke from the cigarettes according to a standardized puffing procedure. Each dose was presented to each subject on four different occasions. Self-reported (subjective), observer-reported (behavioral), and physiologic variables were measured before, during, and after drug administration. The functional equivalence of intravenous nicotine to tobacco smoke was shown by the finding that nicotine produced a similar profile of effects across a variety of measures when given intravenously or by smoke inhalation (Fig. 1). Furthermore, the reliable discriminations of nicotine from placebo were consistent with the fact that nicotine is psychoactive. Its self-reported effects peaked within 1 min after administration (by either route) and dissipated within a few minutes; the peak and duration of

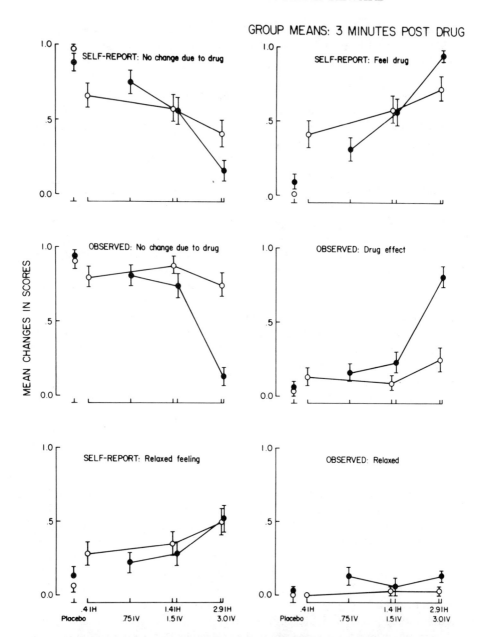

FIG. 1. Summary of change from baseline scores on instruments for measuring self-reported and observer-reported changes. Measures were taken immediately before and about 3 min following drug administration (*N* = 32; 8 subjects × 4 sessions). *Open circles,* inhaled (IH) nicotine; *closed circles,* intravenous (IV) nicotine. (From Henningfield et al., ref. 28, with permission.)

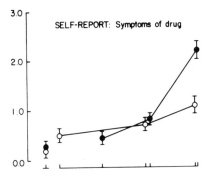

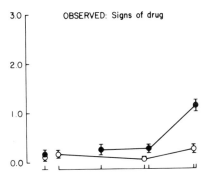

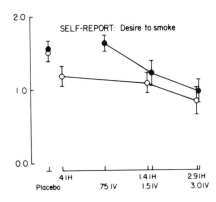

FIG. 1. (Continued)

responses were directly related to the dose. The two indicators of euphoria used
in these studies were the Liking Scale (Single Dose Questionnaire) and the Morphine Benzedrine Group (MBG) Scale of the Addiction Research Center Inventory (ARCI) (37). Figure 2 shows responses on the 5-point Liking Scale, which
asked how much the drug was liked (0, "not at all;" 4, "an awful lot"). Nicotine

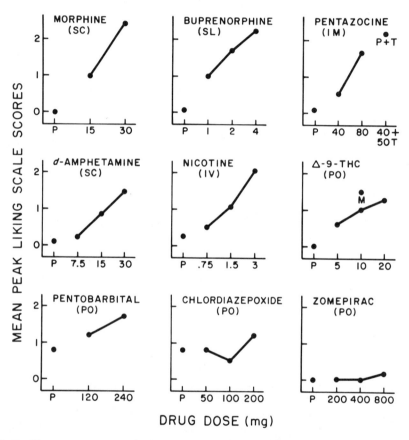

FIG. 2. Mean scores on the "Liking" scale of the Single Dose Questionnaire from subjects
tested at the Addiction Research Center show that nicotine is similar to other drugs of abuse on
this measure. The number of subjects in each group range from 6 (pentobarbital and chlordiazepoxide) to 13 (*d*-amphetamine). The high dose of each drug except zomepirac produced significant
($p < 0.05$) increases in scores above placebo data. The responses are peak responses that
occurred after the drug had been given. The time of the peak response ranged from about 1 min
(nicotine) to 5 hr (buprenorphine). Morphine and zomepirac data are from the same group of
subjects as are the pentobarbital and chlordiazepoxide data. The "P + T" point on the pentazocine
graph is the score, by the same subjects, to 40 mg pentazocine given in combination with 50 mg
tripelennamine (an antihistamine that produced a "liking" scale score of 0.9): the street combination
called "T's and Blues's." The "M" point on the δ-9-THC graph is the score, from the same
subjects, obtained after smoking a marijuana cigarette that contained 10 mg (1% by weight)
δ-9-THC. (From Jasinski et al., ref. 37, with permission.)

produced responses that were similar to those of more commonly studied drugs of abuse, such as morphine and *d*-amphetamine. Scores on the MBG scale of the ARCI were consistent with the Liking Scale data, confirming that nicotine was a euphoriant. When asked to identify the injections from a list of commonly used and abused drugs, subjects frequently identified nicotine injections as cocaine.

Similar physiological effects, including changes in pupil diameter, blood pressure, and skin temperature, were obtained when nicotine was administered intravenously, as well as by inhalation. These similarities in subjective and physiologic responses to nicotine given as either tobacco smoke or intravenous nicotine indicated that nicotine was the active constituent that accounted for these effects of tobacco smoke. A subsequent study showed that nicotine's subjective and physiological effects could be blocked partially by pretreating the subjects with mecamylamine (29). The results of these studies were analogous to those obtained in animal discrimination studies (45,51).

Abuse Liability Studies of Nicotine: Self-Administration

A second type of abuse liability study involves the assessment of the conditions under which an animal or human subject will voluntarily take the substance and thereby determines whether the drug will serve as a positive reinforcer. Variants of this strategy may be conducted using either animals or human subjects, providing a means of establishing the generality of the phenomena while controlling the possible confounding influence of personality, social, or cultural variables. A high degree of concordance between findings from animal and human studies has been established over a wide range of drugs (16,17,47). Studies of nicotine self-administration using animals have shown that nicotine, under a variety of conditions, can serve as a reinforcer for five species (cf. ref. 24). The section below focuses on the results from studies using human volunteers.

In one study (27), 6 volunteers were tested during 3-hr sessions in which 10 presses on a lever resulted in either a nicotine or placebo injection. The subjects were not permitted to smoke cigarettes for 1 hr before or during the study. The main finding was that all of the subjects voluntarily self-administered nicotine. Patterns of self-administration were similar to those observed when human subjects smoked cigarettes and when rhesus monkeys worked (e.g., pressed a lever) to produce intravenous amphetamine injections in comparable experimental situations (17).

In one of the subjects, the pattern of acquisition of nicotine self-administration developed gradually, over several sessions, and double-blind substitution of saline for nicotine resulted in extinction of the self-injection behavior (Fig. 3). Another study (23) showed that when subjects were given simultaneous access to both nicotine and placebo (by pressing alternate levers), they chose nicotine, confirming that nicotine had come to serve as a positive reinforcer.

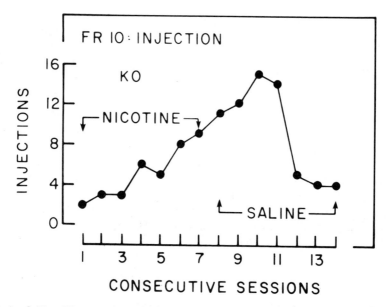

FIG. 3. Subject KO was a cigarette smoker without a history of drug abuse. Ten lever-presses on one lever resulted in delivery of either saline or nicotine; pressing the other lever had no programmed consequence. Nicotine was available (1.5 mg nicotine per injection) during seven consecutive sessions; then saline was substituted for seven additional sessions. Numbers of injections per session are shown on the x-axis. (From Henningfield and Goldberg, ref. 23, with permission.)

Implications of Abuse Liability Studies

The results of these studies provide direct evidence that nicotine itself, apart from its being presented in combination with all of the sensory properties of tobacco smoke, is a drug that can act as a euphoriant and a reinforcer. Thus, nicotine meets the critical criteria of an abusable drug: it is psychoactive, produces euphoria, and serves as a reinforcer. For animals, the conditions under which nicotine serves as a reinforcer are more restricted than with morphine or cocaine. This fact suggests that nicotine self-administration, in the form of tobacco smoke inhalation or smokeless tobacco use, provides ideal confluences of conditions for the establishment and maintenance of nicotine dependence in humans (21), since peripheral taste and olfactory stimuli provided by tobacco products are immediate and abundant. Supporting this line of reasoning, the animal studies that have demonstrated the most robust reinforcing properties of nicotine were those in which nicotine injections were paired with discrete environmental cues, for which, in turn, the animals voluntarily worked, suggesting that ancillary stimuli were important in establishing compulsive-appearing behavior (14,15).

Physical Dependence Potential of Nicotine

Administration of many drugs of abuse results in neuroadaptation, which is measured by tolerance to the repeated administration of the drug and a subsequent rebound (withdrawal phenomena) when drug administration is terminated (32). Tolerance to drug effects is determined either by the diminished response to repeated doses of a drug or the requirement of increasing doses to achieve the same response. Tolerance to the behavioral and physiological effects of nicotine have been studied (cf. ref. 22). As is the case with other drugs of abuse, a variety of mechanisms account for tolerance to many of nicotine's effects. They include metabolic (3), behavioral (6,50,52), and physiologic tolerance (9,12,13). More recent studies have shown that subjective effects of nicotine also show tolerance with repeated dosing (21,38).

Physical dependence (neuroadaptation) is determined by showing that termination of drug administration produces a syndrome of effects, generally opposite in direction of those produced by drug administration and that this syndrome is reversible (at least in its early stages) by administration of the drug for those effects that are true withdrawal effects; prolonged drug abstinence results in eventual return to baseline values of behavioral and physiological functions. Nicotine produces physical dependence, and some of the recent relevant findings will be summarized below.

One series of studies that strongly suggested that tobacco withdrawal was specifically due to nicotine were those of Fagerstrom (10,11), who developed a psychometric instrument (Fagerstrom Tolerance Questionnaire) that could predict which tobacco users would show physical dependence on nicotine and which would be most efficaciously treated using a nicotine substitution procedure (nicotine gum). However, the conditions leading to physical dependence were not clear. For instance, the specific role of preabstinence nicotine intake, the possible ancillary role of other tobacco constituents (e.g., CO and CO_2 in tobacco smoke), and species differences remained in question. A more recent series of studies (19,20,30) conducted at the University of Minnesota have helped to resolve several earlier points of controversy; the results are summarized below.

Three studies evaluated the physical dependence potential of nicotine and established the reliability of various measures of withdrawal. In one of these studies (20), 27 smokers resided for 7 days on a research ward. Following baseline measurements, they either abstained from smoking or continued smoking for 4 days. A battery of physiological, subjective, and behavioral measures were obtained and analyzed. A second study was conducted on a nonresidential basis to assess tobacco withdrawal in a nonlaboratory environment (30). Signs and symptoms of tobacco withdrawal were measured in 100 smokers. Following baseline measurements, subjects were randomly assigned to groups that received either nicotine or placebo gum, which was to be chewed at their own rate. The subjects returned on three different occasions for assessment. The third study

(19) assessed the reliability of the tobacco withdrawal syndrome within subjects. This study employed a modified within-subject experimental design (baseline smoking, tobacco deprivation, return to baseline smoking, and tobacco deprivation assessed in each subject).

These studies demonstrated that the withdrawal syndrome that occurs reliably and consistently in chronic smokers after tobacco deprivation includes the following effects: (a) decreased heart rate, (b) increased caloric intake/eating, (c) increased number of awakenings from sleep, (d) increased desire to smoke cigarettes, and (e) impatience and confusion. Other changes that occurred in some of the studies included increased irritability and decreased vigor. A prospective examination of data revealed that there were no statistically significant differences between men and women regarding the number or severity of tobacco withdrawal symptoms (53). Two subsequent investigations extended the generality of conditions under which nicotine withdrawal may occur. One of these showed that smokeless forms of tobacco may produce physical dependence (18), and the other showed that nicotine gum may produce physiological dependence (31). More recently, results from a nicotine physical dependence study at the Addiction Research Center showed that the tobacco withdrawal syndrome includes reliable deficits in cognitive performance that are associated with changes in electrophysiological measures of brain function and that these effects are reversible in a dose-related fashion by nicotine gum. Additional results from this study are consistent with those described above (19,20,30).

Implications of Physical Dependence Potential Studies

The aforementioned studies confirm and extend previous findings that nicotine has the potential to produce physical dependence. It is now clear that the tobacco abstinence syndrome results from the administration and withdrawal of nicotine. Its overt signs are less dramatic than those that mark opioid and sedative withdrawal, but they are not necessarily less important to the individual. For instance, withdrawal effects such as mood changes, performance deficits, and weight gain are of considerable potential disruption to normal functioning. The next section reviews autoradiographic data demonstrating that systemic nicotine administration results in the distribution of nicotine to the brain, that nicotine is localized to specific binding sites in the brain, and that nicotine alters cerebral function, as evidenced by effects on cerebral glucose utilization.

AUTORADIOGRAPHIC STUDIES OF REGIONAL DISTRIBUTION, RECEPTOR BINDING, AND CEREBRAL METABOLIC EFFECTS OF NICOTINE

Schmiterlow and colleagues made a number of important observations during the 1950s and 1960s that provided one of the cornerstones upon which the role of nicotine in tobacco dependence was formulated. They used radiotracer techniques and found that nicotine accumulated in the CNS following administration by various routes (intramuscular, subcutaneous, intravenous). More recent technical developments in the area of receptor pharmacology led to studies on the *in vitro* specific binding of radiolabelled nicotine to brain homogenates or slide-mounted brain sections. The radioligand used most often was racemic tritiated nicotine, although the tritiated *l*-isomer has become available recently. Specific binding is defined as the radioactivity that is displaced by a saturating concentration of ligand. In studies of [³H]nicotine receptor binding, nonspecific and specific (total minus nonspecific) binding have been determined using unlabelled nicotine, *d*-tubocurarine, and hexamethonium as the displacers. Early studies of the cerebral distribution of specific [³H]nicotine binding sites were performed on synaptosomal or crude membrane preparations from regions of rat or mouse brain (41,42,57). More recently, regional specific binding of [³H]nicotine has been demonstrated (7) and quantitated (40) in the rat brain using light microscopic autoradiography.

London and her colleagues showed that [³H]nicotine binding was heterogeneously distributed throughout the brain, with the densest labeling in the interpeduncular nucleus and medial habenula (Table 2). Dense to intermediate levels of labeling also were seen in the superior colliculus, thalamic nuclei, and the cerebral cortex. In the hippocampal formation, a slightly lower level of specific binding was localized to the subiculum and the molecular layer of the dentate gyrus. Labeling in the caudate-putamen and the hypothalamus was sparse, and there was no significant specific binding in the hilus of the dentate gyrus, in the CA1 subfield of Ammon's horn, or in the periaqueductal gray matter.

TABLE 2. *Densities of [³H]nicotine binding sites in selected brain regions*[a]

Brain region	Density of sites (fmol/mg tissue)
Parietal cortex, layer IV	8.4 ± 0.3
Caudate putamen	1.7 ± 0.4
Hypothalamus, posterior nucleus	1.8 ± 0.4
Thalamus, ventral posterior nucleus	11 ± 2.2
Lateral geniculate body, dorsal	5.8 ± 0.7
Accessory optic nucleus	5.1 ± 0.6
Medial geniculate body	4.8 ± 1.0
Superior colliculus	13 ± 0.6
Interpeduncular nucleus	28 ± 2.0
Medial habenula	26 ± 1.8
Dentate gyrus, molecular layer	3.2 ± 0.8

[a] Results are expressed as the means ($\pm$SE) for 40–48 measurements per region (10–12 readings per area from 4 rats). The density of sites was taken as the difference between total binding and nonspecific binding determined in the absence or presence of 1 mM unlabeled *l*-nicotine, respectively.
Data from London et al. (40).

Although specific binding may indicate the presence of true functional receptors, this condition does not always hold. Furthermore, because the brain is a highly interconnected organ, drugs may produce effects in brain regions remote from their initial receptor interactions. For this reason, an *in vivo* functional mapping procedure could provide additional information about the distribution of nicotine's effects in the brain. The autoradiographic 2-deoxy-D-[1-^{14}C]glucose (2-DG) method (49) measures local cerebral glucose utilization (LCGU) and has been used to demonstrate a close relation between local cerebral function and glucose utilization under a wide variety of experimental conditions (48). This method was used to measure the *in vivo* effects of nicotine on LCGU, and the pattern of LCGU was compared with the reported distributions of [^{3}H]nicotine binding (39).

In these studies, nicotine stimulated LCGU in specific brain regions (Table 3). The greatest increase occurred in the medial habenula. Marked increases were noted in the anteroventral thalamic nucleus, interpeduncular nucleus, and superior colliculus. Moderate increases were seen in the retrosplenial cortex, interanteromedial thalamic nucleus, and lateral geniculate body. No significant effects were observed in the frontoparietal cortex, lateral habenula, or central gray matter. LCGU responses to nicotine were completely blocked by mecamylamine (data not shown), indicating specificity of nicotine's effects.

The findings correlated well with the distributions of [^{3}H]nicotine binding sites (7,39). Those areas, such as thalamic nuclei, the interpeduncular nucleus, medial habenula, and the superior colliculus, that showed dense labelling with [^{3}H]nicotine also manifested moderate to marked nicotine-induced LCGU increases. Areas with less specific binding showed lesser LCGU responses to nicotine, and the central gray matter, which lacked specific [^{3}H]nicotine binding,

TABLE 3. *Effects of d,1-nicotine on glucose utilization in the rat brain*[a]

Brain region	Local cerebral glucose utilization (μmol/100 g tissue/min)	
	Saline control	Nicotine (1.75 mg/kg)
Frontoparietal cortex, layer IV	110 ± 8.1	108 ± 6.5
Retrosplenial cortex, layer I	98 ± 6.5	123 ± 5.1[b]
Thalamic nuclei		
Anteroventral	109 ± 6.5	201 ± 6.1[b]
Interanteromedial	125 ± 8.6	175 ± 12.3[b]
Lateral geniculate body	82 ± 6.8	106 ± 4.4[b]
Interpeduncular nucleus	99 ± 9.8	182 ± 9.3[b]
Medial Habenula	70 ± 7.0	167 ± 3.7[b]
Superior colliculus	72 ± 5.2	142 ± 4.6[b]
Central grey matter	66 ± 4.0	77 ± 4.3

[a] Results are expressed as the mean ± SE for 4 rats per group.
[b] Significantly different from saline control, $p < 0.05$.

demonstrated no LCGU response. Similarly, nicotine dramatically increased LCGU in the medial but not the lateral habenula, reflecting densities of [^{3}H]nicotine binding sites. An inconsistency was observed in the neocortex, where layer IV showed significant [^{3}H]nicotine binding but no LCGU response to nicotine. These results suggested that [^{3}H]nicotine binding sites visualized autoradiographically in the rat brain are functional nicotine receptors. The demonstration of specific receptors for nicotine may open the way to the development of new means to intervene in nicotine dependence or to the development of less toxic substances that retain some of nicotine's more useful actions.

CONCLUSIONS

Despite the complexities of tobacco self-administration, systematic analysis has revealed that the resulting dependence process is similar to that produced and maintained by other drugs whose use leads to abuse and physical dependence. Specifically, certain effects of tobacco and the patterns of behavior that result from its use are similar to those produced by drugs that cause abuse and physical dependence. Furthermore, that these effects are due to nicotine itself, which is delivered by all commonly used forms of tobacco, is indicated by the findings that nicotine is psychoactive, produces euphoria, and serves as a reinforcer. Additionally, nicotine has the potential to produce physical dependence and tolerance, and the withdrawal syndrome is alleviated by nicotine administration. Together, these characteristics of nicotine distinguish it as a drug with a considerable potential to control the behavior of people who use tobacco (i.e., cause drug dependence). Progress in identifying neurobiological correlates of nicotine's effects have also been made, as described in the present paper. These findings have implications for public health policy, which now widely acknowledges that tobacco is appropriately categorized as an addictive or dependence-producing drug (cf., refs. 44, 49, 55, and 56).

REFERENCES

1. American Hospital Formulary Services (1984): *Drug Information Supplement B,* pp. 39B–44B. American Society of Hospital Pharmaceuticals, Bethesda, Maryland.
2. Austin, G. A. (1978): *Perspectives on the History of Psychoactive Substance Use. National Institute on Drug Abuse Research Monograph 24.* U.S. Government Printing Office, Washington, D.C.
3. Beckett, A. H., and Triggs, E. J. (1967): Enzyme induction in man caused by smoking. *Nature,* 216:587.
4. Brady, J. V., and Lukas, S. E., editors (1984): *Testing Drugs for Physical Dependence Potential and Abuse Liability. National Institute on Drug Abuse Research Monograph 52.* U.S. Government Printing Office, Washington, D.C.
5. Brecker, E. M., and the Editors of Consumers Union Reports (1972): *Licit and Illicit Drugs.* Little, Brown and Company, Boston.
6. Clarke, P. B. S., and Kumar, R. (1983): The effects of nicotine on locomotor activity in nontolerant and tolerant rats. *Br. J. Pharmacol.,* 78:239–337.
7. Clarke, P. B. S., Pert, C. B., and Pert A. (1984): Autoradiographic distribution of nicotine receptors in rat brain. *Brain Res.,* 323:390–395.

8. Connolly, G. N., Winn, D. M., Hecht, S. S., Henningfield, J. E., Hoffman, D., and Walker, B. (1986): Science public policy and the re-emergence of smokeless tobacco. *N. Engl. J. Med.,* 314: 1020–1027.
9. Domino, E. F. (1979): Behavioral, electrophysiological, endocrine and skeletal muscle actions of nicotine and tobacco smoking. In: *Electrophysiological Effects of Nicotine,* edited by A. Remond and C. Izard, pp. 133–146. Elsevier, Amsterdam.
10. Fagerstrom, K. (1978): Measuring degree of physical dependence to tobacco smoking with reference to individualization to treatment. *Addict. Behav.,* 3:235–241.
11. Fagerstrom, K. (1981): Tobacco smoking, nicotine dependence and smoking cessation. Doctoral thesis. Uppsala University, Uppsala, Sweden.
12. Fagerstrom, K. O., and Gotestam, K. G. (1977): Increase in muscle tonus after tobacco smoking. *Addict. Behav.,* 2:203–206.
13. Faulkerborn, Y., Larsson, C., and Nordberg, A. (1981): Chronic nicotine exposure in rat: A behavioural and biochemical study of tolerance. *Drug Alcohol Depend.,* 8:51–60.
14. Goldberg, S. R., and Spealman, R. D. (1982): Maintenance and suppression of behavior by intravenous nicotine injections in squirrel monkeys. *Fed. Proc.,* 41:216–220.
15. Goldberg, S. R., Spealman, R. D., and Goldberg, D. M. (1981): Persistent behavior at high rates maintained by intravenous self-administration of nicotine. *Science,* 214:573–575.
16. Griffiths, R. R., and Balster, R. L. (1979): Opioids: Similarity between evaluations of subjective effects and animal self-administration results. *Clin. Pharmacol. Ther.,* 25:611–617.
17. Griffiths, R. R., Bigelow, G. E., and Henningfield, J. E. (1980): Similarities in animal and human drug taking behavior. In: *Advances in Substance Abuse: Behavioral and Biological Research,* edited by N. K. Mellow, pp. 1–90. JAI Press, Greenwich, Connecticut.
18. Hatsukami, D. K., Gust, S. W., and Keenan, R. (1986): Physiological and subjective changes from smokeless tobacco withdrawal. *Clin. Pharmacol. Ther.,* (*in press*).
19. Hatsukami, D. K., Hughes, J. R., and Pickens, R. W. (1985): Characteristics of tobacco abstinence: Physiological and subjective effects. In: *Pharmacological Adjuncts in Smoking Cessation. National Institute on Drug Abuse Research Monograph 53,* edited by J. Grabowski and S. M. Hall, pp. 56–67. U.S. Government Printing Office, Washington, D.C.
20. Hatsukami, D. K., Hughes, J. R., Pickens, R. W., and Svikis, D. (1984): Tobacco withdrawal symptoms: An experimental analysis. *Psychopharmacology (Berlin),* 84:231–236.
21. Henningfield, J. E. (1984): Behavioral pharmacology of cigarette smoking. In: *Advances in Behavioral Pharmacology, Vol. 4,* edited by T. Thompson, P. B. Dews, and J. E. Barrett, pp. 131–210. Academic Press, Orlando.
22. Henningfield, J. E. (1984): Pharmacologic basis and treatment of cigarette smoking. *J. Clin. Psychiatry,* 45:24–34.
23. Henningfield, J. E., and Goldberg, S. R. (1983): Control of behavior by intravenous nicotine injections in human subjects. *Pharmacol. Biochem. Behav.,* 19:1021–1026.
24. Henningfield, J. E., and Goldberg, S. R. (1983): Nicotine as a reinforcer in human subjects and laboratory animals. *Pharmacol. Biochem. Behav.,* 19:989–992.
25. Henningfield, J. E., Griffiths, R. R., and Jasinski, D. R. (1981): Human dependence on tobacco and opioids: Common factors. In: *Behavioral Pharmacology of Human Drug Dependence. National Institute on Drug Abuse Research Monograph 37,* edited by T. Thompson and C. E. Johanson, pp. 210–234. U.S. Government Printing Office, Washington, D.C.
26. Henningfield, J. E., Lukas, S. E., and Bigelow, G. E. (1986): Human studies of drugs as reinforcers. In: *Behavioral Analysis of Drug Dependence,* edited by S. R. Goldberg and I. P. Stolerman, pp. 69–122. Academic Press, New York.
27. Henningfield, J. E., Miyasato, K., and Jasinski, D. R. (1983): Cigarette smokers self-administer intravenous nicotine. *Pharmacol. Biochem. Behav.,* 19:887–890.
28. Henningfield, J. E., Miyasato, K., and Jasinksi, D. R. (1985): Abuse liability and pharmacodynamic characteristics of intravenous and inhaled nicotine. *J. Pharmacol. Exp. Ther.,* 234:1–12.
29. Henningfield, J. E., Miyasato, K., Johnson, R. E., and Jasinski, D. R. (1983): Rapid physiologic effects of nicotine in humans and selective blockade of behavioral effects by mecamylamine. *Problems of Drug Dependence. National Institute on Drug Abuse Research Monograph 43.* U.S. Government Printing Office, Washington, D.C.
30. Hughes, J. R., and Hatsukami, D. (1986): Signs and symptoms of tobacco withdrawal. *Arch. Gen. Psychiatry,* 43:289–295.
31. Hughes, J. R., Hatsukami, D., and Skoog, K. P. (1986): Physical dependence on nicotine gum: A placebo substitution trial. *J.A.M.A.,* 255:3277–3279.

32. Jaffe, J. H. (1985): Drug addiction and drug abuse. In: *Goodman and Gillman's The Pharmacological Basis of Therapeutics,* edited by A. G. Gilman, L. S. Goodman, T. W. Rall, and F. Murad, pp. 532–581. Macmillan, New York.
33. Jaffe, J. H., and Kanzler, M. (1979): Smoking as an addictive disorder. In: *Cigarette Smoking as a Dependence Process. National Institute on Drug Abuse Research Monograph 23,* edited by N. A. Krasnegor, pp. 4–23. U.S. Government Printing Office, Washington, D.C.
34. Jarvik, M. (1970): The role of nicotine in the smoking habit. In: *Learning Mechanisms in Smoking,* edited by W. A. Hunt, pp. 155–190. Aldine, Chicago.
35. Jarvik, M. (1973): Further observations on nicotine as the reinforcing agent in smoking. In: *Smoking Behavior: Motives and Incentives,* edited by W. L. Dunn, pp. 33–49. Winston, Washington, D.C.
36. Jasinski, D. R. (1977): Assessment of the abuse potential of morphine-like drugs (methods used in man). In: *Handbook of Experimental Pharmacology,* edited by W. R. Martin, pp. 197–258. Springer-Verlag, Heidelberg, Federal Republic of Germany.
37. Jasinski, D. R., Johnson, R. E., and Henningfield, J. E. (1984): Abuse liability assessment in human subjects. *Trends Pharmacol. Sci.,* 5:196–200.
38. Jones, R. T., Farrell, T. R., and Herning, R. I. (1978): Tobacco smoking and nicotine tolerance. In: *Self-Administration of Abused Substances: Methods for Study. National Institute on Drug Abuse Research Monograph 20,* pp. 202–208. U.S. Government Printing Office, Washington, D.C.
39. London, E. D., Connolly, R. J., Szikszay, M., and Wamsley, J. K. (1985): Distribution of cerebral metabolic effects of nicotine in the rat. *Eur. J. Pharmacol.,* 110:391–392.
40. London, E. D., Waller, S. B., and Wamsley, J. K. (1985): Autoradiographic localization of [^{3}H]nicotine binding sites in the rat brain. *Neurosci. Lett.,* 53:179–184.
41. Marks, M. J., and Collins, A. C. (1982): Characterization of nicotine binding in mouse brain and comparison with binding of bungarotoxin and quinuclidinyl benzilate. *Mol. Pharmacol.,* 22:554–564.
42. Martin, B. R., and Aceto, M. D. (1981): Nicotine binding sites and their localization in the central nervous system. *Neurosci. Behav. Rev.,* 5:473–478.
43. Martin, W. R. (1977): In: *Handbook of Experimental Pharmacology: Vol. 45, Drug Addiction I,* edited by W. R. Martin, pp. 3–42. Springer-Verlag, Berlin, Heidelberg.
44. Pollin, W. (1984): The role of the addictive process as a key step in causation of all tobacco-related diseases. *J.A.M.A.,* 252:2874.
45. Rosecrans, J. A. (1986): Brain area cites of nicotine action: Evidence for noncholinergic mechanisms. *Proceedings of the International Symposium on Tobacco Smoking and Health: A Neurobiological Approach (in press).*
46. Russell, M. A. H. (1971): Cigarette smoking: National history of a dependence disorder. *Br. J. Med. Psychol.,* 44:1–16.
47. Schuster, C. R., and Johanson, C. E. (1985): Efficacy, dependence potential, and neurotoxicity of anorectic drugs. In: *Behavioral Pharmacology: The Current Status,* edited by L. S. Seiden and R. L. Balster, pp. 263–279. Alan R. Liss, New York.
48. Sokoloff, L. (1981): Localization of functional activity in the central nervous system by measurement activity of glucose utilization with radioactive deoxyglucose. *J. Cereb. Blood Flow Metab.,* 1:7–36.
49. Sokoloff, L., Reivich, M., Kennedy, C., Des Rosiers, M. H., Patlak, C. S., Petigrew, K. D., Sakurada, O., and Shinohara, M. (1977): The ^{14}C-deoxyglucose method for the measurement of local cerebral glucose utilization: Theory, procedure, and normal values in the conscious and anesthetized albino rat. *J. Neurochem.,* 28:897.
50. Stitzer, M., Morrison, J., and Domino, E. F. (1970): Effects of nicotine on fixed-interval behavior and their modification by cholinergic antagonists. *J. Pharmacol. Exp. Ther.,* 171:166–177.
51. Stolerman, I. P. (1986): Discriminative stimulus properties in nicotine: Correlations with nicotine binding. *Proceedings of the International Symposium on Tobacco Smoking and Health: A Neurobiologic Approach (in press).*
52. Stolerman, I. P., Bunker, P., and Jarvik, M. E. (1974): Nicotine tolerance in rats: Role of dose and dose interval. *Psychopharmacology (Berlin),* 34:317–324.
53. Svikis, D. S., Hatsukami, D. K., Hughs, J. R., Carroll, K. M., and Pickens, R. W. (1986): Sex differences in tobacco withdrawal syndrome. *Addict. Behav. (in press).*
54. U.S. Department of Health, Education and Welfare (1979): *Smoking and Health: A Report of the Surgeon General.* U.S. Government Printing Office, Washington, D.C.

55. U.S. Department of Health and Human Services (1984): *Drug Abuse and Drug Abuse Research. The First in a Series of Triennial Reports to Congress,* pp. 85–104. U.S. Government Printing Office, Washington, D.C.
56. U.S. Department of Health and Human Services, Public Health Service (1983): *Why People Smoke Cigarettes* (PHS Publication No. PHS 83-50195). U.S. Government Printing Office, Washington, D.C.
57. Yoshida, K., and Imura, H. (1979): Nicotine cholinergic receptors in brain synaptosomes. *Brain Res.,* 172:453–459.
58. Wesnes, K., and Warburton, D. M. (1982): Smoking, nicotine and human performance. *Pharmacol. Ther.,* 21:189–234.
59. Wesnes, K., and Warburton, D. M. (1983): Smoking, nicotine and human performance. *Pharmacol. Ther.,* 21:189–208.
60. Wesnes, K., and Warburton, D. M. (1984): The effects of cigarettes varying yield on rapid information processing performance. *Psychopharmacology (Berlin),* 82:338–342.
61. World Health Organization (1981): Nomenclature and classification of drug- and alcohol-related problems: A WHO Memorandum. *Bull. WHO,* 59:225–242.

Brain Reward Systems and Abuse, edited by
J. Engel and L. Oreland.
Raven Press, New York © 1987.

Biological Connection Between Sensation Seeking and Drug Abuse

Marvin Zuckerman

Department of Psychology, University of Delaware, Newark, Delaware 19716

For a full understanding of drug abuse we must investigate (a) the subjective motivations of the drug abuser; (b) the basic personality of the drug abuser and the related motivational traits; (c) the biological effects of the abused drugs in the nervous system with specific interest in their effects on reward systems; (d) the specific biological characteristics of drug abusers that may be relevant to their vulnerability to the effects of the drug; (e) the broader social reinforcements involved in the drug life and how they interact with the personality and motivations of the drug abuser. I intend to look at all of these questions with a somewhat myopic view through the trait and motive called "sensation seeking."

SUBJECTIVE MOTIVATIONS OF THE DRUG ABUSER

The most frequent reasons given by college students for using marijuana, LSD and other hallucinogens, depressants, and narcotics (38) are "to experience something new and different" or "curiosity." The principle reason for using stimulants is "energy," and new experience is a close second. Sociability is given as the primary reason for using alcohol. Most of these college students were probably not drug-dependent, and the search for novel experience would probably not characterize the heavy drug abuser dependent on a specific drug. In such individuals, the primary reason for use may be either an attempt to recreate the euphoria produced by the drug before they developed a tolerance, or to avoid the psychological or physiological pain of withdrawal. However, it is clear that in the early stages the drug user is looking for some kind of reward that is outside of the realm of natural experiences. This is not to say that drugs provide the only rewards for users or abusers. Zuckerman et al. (50) found that sexual experience among both male and female college students was positively correlated with drug experience. In the several years I worked with drug abusers in a therapeutic community, I discovered that their social, sexual, and even criminal activities also provided rewards that reinforced the use of drugs. I still hear psychodynamic conceptions that imply that the primary reason for abuse of drugs

165

is an attempt to narcotize anxiety or depression. Segal et al. (38) found this reason given by only 6 to 12% of drug users for all drugs except depressants (alcohol, barbiturates, tranquilizers), where 21% gave this reason. My experience with community drug abusers suggested that anxiety or depression were quite rare in this group other than dysphoric feelings engendered by life circumstances like getting arrested or not being able to get their drugs.

PERSONALITY OF THE DRUG ABUSER

The general definition of sensation seeking as "the need for varied, novel, and complex sensations and experiences and the willingness to take physical and social risks for the sake of such experience" (46) explains why this trait has been the one most highly related to drug use and abuse. If we consider the basic four sensation-seeking factors, embodied in the scales of forms IV and V (51) of the Sensation Seeking Scales (SSS), we can see how drugs and the drug life can satisfy the general motive and its specific forms of expression.

Thrill and Adventure Seeking

Thrill- and adventure-seeking (TAS) is satisfied by the risks of the criminal activities that are involved in the use, buying, and selling of illegal drugs. It also explains why the sensation-seeking drug abuser is not deterred by the physical dangers involved in the use of potentially lethal drugs.

Experience Seeking

Experience-seeking (ES) is most satisfied by psychedelic drugs where the effects are least predictable from one occasion to the next. However, stimulants are also used to enhance other types of experience such as those involved in social and sexual interactions.

Disinhibition

Disinhibition (Dis) provides an explanation for the attraction of alcohol and other depressants. Alcohol has been essential to parties, feasts, carnivals, and orgies, in general, since the beginning of civilization and probably before then. Disinhibition describes both a psychological-behavioral and a physiological phenomenon, since alcohol acts first on brain centers that are inhibitory, thus disinhibiting the systems they regulate. The strange thing is that the persons most attracted to alcohol and other depressants are those who are least inhibited prior to taking the drug.

Boredom Susceptibility

Boredom susceptibility (BS) describes the vulnerability of the sensation-seeker to conditions where there is no variety in stimulation from tasks or other persons. All drugs have been used to deal with boredom. The typical 9-to-5 job, whether manual or clerical, seldom provides enough stimulation for the high-sensation-seeker and constitutes 8 hr of aversive conditions, which the sensation-seeker tries to compensate for by using drugs or alcohol off and, too often, on the job as well.

Given the relevance of the sensation-seeking motive to drug use, it is not surprising that many studies (46,47) have shown this personality trait to be the one most highly related to drug use among college students (38), sailors (38), soldiers (19), veterans (16), and members of labor unions (15). SSS scores are related more to the variety and extent of drug use than to use of any specific drug, although stimulant and hallucinogenic drug users seem to be somewhat higher on the trait than primarily depressant or opiate users (5,39). However, comparing young heroin users with their delinquent peers (31), it is apparent that they are also high sensation-seekers. In a paper presented at a recent meeting at the National Institute of Drug Abuse, Craig (7) described heroin addicts in the following terms: "They cannot tolerate boredom, are playful, want change, are exhibitionistic, high in sensation seeking and are stimulus augmenters rather than stimulus reducers."

While drug abusers are higher than exclusively alcohol abusers on sensation-seeking (16,38), sensation-seeking is positively related to extent of alcohol use in college students (37), soldiers (19), and in alcoholics (17,24), where the more chronic types tend to be higher than the more acute and later developing types. Apparently, years of alcohol use do not dampen sensation-seeking needs.

Apart from sensation-seeking, Craig (7) has described heroin addicts as having traits typical of "traditional anti-social psychopathy," including hostility, immaturity, impulsiveness, a low tolerance for frustration, high sexual needs, and low needs for endurance and affiliation. In a study of residents in a therapeutic community for drug abusers, we (52) found that about two-thirds of the males and over 90% of the females showed the typical psychopathic profile on the Minnesota Multiphasic Personality Inventory (MMPI) after about 6 months of drug-free time in the treatment facility. Primary psychopaths, as opposed to secondary psychopaths and nonpsychopathic criminals, score high on the SSS, particularly the Disinhibition subscale (4,10). While psychopaths are sensation-seekers, most high sensation seekers are not psychopaths. Nonpsychopathic high sensation seekers may have empathy for others and find outlets for their sensation seeking needs that are not antisocial.

EFFECTS OF DRUGS ON BRAIN REWARD SYSTEMS

There is a danger in theorizing in areas that are far from one's own area of expertise. In 1978, while writing my book on sensation seeking (46), I discovered

Stein's (41) model relating the catecholamine systems to the reward effects produced by self-stimulation. Although aware that Stein's view of the primary involvement of the dorsal noradrenergic bundle and the locus ceruleus in positive reinforcement had not gone unchallenged, I made it the basis of a biological model of sensation-seeking. The evidence for the catecholamine basis of reward stemmed largely from studies of intracranial self-stimulation behavior and self-injections of catecholamine releasors like amphetamine and cocaine in rats, monkeys, and humans. These studies suggest that there must be more than human social factors or the search for novel experience involved in drug abuse. The stimulant drugs seem to activate primary reward centers in the brain, thus providing a pleasurable hedonic experience. However, work with more selective blockers and depletors of norepinephrine has shown that while dopamine is essential for the phenomena in some brain sites, norepinephrine is not (25,44). New evidence (6) also suggests that self-stimulation may be obtained from areas like the thalamus that are not rich in either catecholamine. By the time of my 1984 paper (48), I shifted to the view that the noradrenergic system was primarily an arousal one, responsive to novel stimuli and positively reinforcing only at moderate levels of activity. While dopaminergic systems may be primarily responsible for intrinsic brain reward, they also show reversals of effects as a function of dosage of stimulant drug agonists (9). The euphoria, socialization, and high activity produced by amphetamine, for instance, may give way to anxiety, withdrawal, and stereotyped and repetitive activity at high doses reached as a function of tolerance. The mechanisms for these reversals are not understood, but they could be due to depletion, the destruction of receptors, or the activation of negative feedback mechanisms.

Stein (41) had also proposed that endorphins might provide another type of positive reinforcement related to drive reduction and that opiate drugs may be rewarding because of their effects on these receptors. However, Wise (44,45) has suggested that opiates, like stimulants, may provide reward and pleasure through their actions on dopamine systems. Dworkin and Smith (8) found that self-administered morphine in rats increased dopamine and norepinephrine turnover in some brain sites, while reducing the activity of the catecholamines in other sites. The drug LSD also has been shown to increase dopaminergic activity, while decreasing noradrenergic activity (12). Alcohol increases synthesis and turnover for all monoamine systems, although it may block receptors for norepinephrine (27). While the psychopharmacological identification of reward systems is far from complete, it is clear that the monoamine systems are involved in the biological mechanisms that support drug use.

MONOAMINES AND SENSATION SEEKING

Little work has been done on the biological characteristics of drug abusers, probably because investigators feel that their systems may have been altered by chronic ingestion of drugs. However, young sensation seekers, who are not yet heavy consumers of drugs but are at risk for drug abuse, might provide a useful group for studying the biological susceptibility to drug addiction.

The first direct connection between the monoamine systems and sensation-seeking trait came from studies of the relationship of the trait to the enzyme monoamine oxidase (MAO) measured in blood platelets. Since the initial studies done at the National Institute of Mental Health (NIMH) (26,36), additional studies have been done in the United States, Sweden, and Spain. Table 1 shows the results of six studies, involving nine groups, that reported correlations between MAO and the General or Total scores on the SSS. Subscales that were significantly correlated with MAO are also listed. All but one of the nine correlations are negative in direction, and six of the nine correlations with General or Total scores were significant. Despite these consistencies in findings there is a large range in the correlation sizes from 0.17 to −0.66. The median correlation was only −0.25. Clearly, there is a significant association between MAO and sensation-seeking, but the reasons for the variability in correlation are not apparent. Sample size may be important, since the smallest significant correlation was found in the largest sample of over 1,000 soldiers (18), and the largest was found in a small sample of only 13 normals (2). However, the first NIMH studies (26,36), finding significant effects in both of two male samples and one of two female samples, used moderate sized Ns but still found fair-sized correlations.

Table 2 shows the correlations between MAO and the Monotony Avoidance scale, which is a short Swedish sensation-seeking scale devised by Schalling et al. (35). In studies (29,30,35) involving three normal groups and three groups of depressed patients, all of the correlations were negative, and three of the six were significant. The median correlation was −0.22, closely resembling that found in the SSS studies.

It is difficult to make inferences about levels of MAO in the central monoaminergic systems or activity of the neurotransmitters in these systems from platelet MAO. However, Adolfsson et al. (1) have found high correlations between MAO

TABLE 1. *Correlations: MAO versus SSS (Gen IV or Total V)*

Authors (reference)	Subjects	N	r	Significant subscales
Murphy et al. (26)	F students	65	0.17	None
	M students	30	−0.45**	Dis
Schooler et al. (36)	F students	47	−0.43**	TAS, ES
	M students	46	−0.52**	TAS, ES, BS
Ballenger et al. (13)	M and F adult	36	−0.17	None (TAS −0.30)
Schalling et al. (35)	M students	40	−0.25	Dis (−0.26*)
von Knorring and Oreland (17)	M soldiers	1129	−0.06*	BS
Arqué et al. (12)	M and F adult	13	−0.66**	TAS, ES, Dis
	M and F patients	44	−0.25*	ES, Dis

* $p < 0.05$; **$p < 0.01$; F, female; M, male; Dis, disinhibition; TAS, thrill- and adventure-seeking; ES, experience-seeking; BS, boredom susceptibility.

TABLE 2. *Correlations: MAO versus monotony avoidance (KSP)*

Authors (reference)	Subjects	N	r
Schalling et al. (35)	M students	40	−0.30*
	M adults	58	−0.16
Fowler et al. (1980)	M and F adults	59	−0.17
Perris et al. (30)	M and F depressed patients	24	−0.55**
Perris et al. (29)	M and F depressed patients	143	−0.18**
	M depressed patients	60	−0.05
	F depressed patients	83	−0.26**

*$p < 0.05$; **$p < 0.01$; M, male; F, female.

activity in different parts of the brain, and Oreland and Fowler (28) have suggested a link between activity in the serotonergic system and MAO. Given the uncertainty about the relationships between the peripheral MAO and the biochemistry of the brain, where the activities occur that govern personality dispositions, it is not surprising that the correlation between any one biological index and personality trait is low. We must also consider the probability that MAO is just one of many biochemical factors involved in the trait. One term in a complex equation cannot predict the solution except within very broad limits. What the MAO data indicate is that we must turn our attention to the monoamine systems as candidates for the biological bases of personality. Until very recently, the only way to study the monoamine brain systems in living humans has been through measuring levels of transmitters, metabolites, and enzymes found in cerebrospinal fluid (CSF), blood, or urine. With the development of neuroselective positon emission tomography (PET) more direct physiological methods will be available. In the meantime, there are only a few correlative studies relating a range of monoamine measures to personality.

Ballenger et al. (3) found negative correlations between plasma dopamine-β-hydroxylase (DBH) and CSF norepinephrine (NE) and sensation-seeking. The negative correlation with DBH was found in two other studies (20,42). Since DBH is the enzyme that converts dopamine to NE in the NE neuron, a low level of DBH in the brain would be consistent with a low level of NE. Schalling et al. (33) measured CSF metabolites of serotonin (5-HIAA), dopamine (HVA), and norepinephrine (MHPG) in a normal group and three patient groups. The serotonin metabolite 5-HIAA correlated negatively with Eysenck and Eysenck's (11) P scale in the normal and two of the patient groups. Recent factor analyses we have conducted using the Karolinska scales along with measures from other widely used tests of basic temperament and personality reveal that the factor marked by the P scale also consists of impulsivity, sensation-seeking, and unsocialized tendencies. Although the Eysencks call this factor "Psychoticism," a better term would be "Psychopathy." Persons scoring high on this factor would be likely to be among those using dangerous and illegal drugs. Low levels of serotonin in high P scorers would be consistent with the clinical data showing a relationship between low serotonin or 5-HIAA levels and violent suicidal or homicidal behavior (22,32). The comparative literature on the effects of serotonin depletion on animal behavior (40) suggest that this system mediates inhibition of behavior and emotional reactions in situations where there is conflict or the possibility of punishment for responding. The association of a deficit in serotonin with impulsive, emotional reactions, and, to some degree, with sensation-seeking in humans, suggests that it is the balance between neurotransmitter systems impelling to action (like dopamine) and those inhibiting action (like serotonin) that influence the relevant personality traits.

A third major study, recently completed in Catalonia, Spain (2), used only indices from blood including plasma MHPG. This measure, also associated with the brain NE system, correlated negatively with Total, ES, and Dis SS scales in a normal group but not in a patient group. While these correlations are consistent with the negative relationship between CSF NE and sensation-seeking in the Ballenger et al. (3) study, that study had also used plasma MHPG and found no relationship between it and sensation-seeking. Two other findings of interest in the Catalonian study were negative correlations between Thyroid Stimulating Hormone (TSH) and SS and between acetylcholinesterase (ACH) and SS in both patient and normal groups. ACH terminates activity in the cholinergic system at the postsynaptic membrane and thus suggests another deficit in neuroregulation that may underlie the trait of sensation seeking.

Since opiate drug abusers are also high-sensation-seekers, it was logical to inquire into the possibility that they were attracted to these drugs because of a deficit in endorphin activity in the brain. Johansson et al. (14) found that chronic pain patients with low levels of fraction I endorphins in CSF were significantly higher on all of the SS scales than those with high levels of endorphins. In the normals studied by Ballenger et al. (3), there were no relationships found between the SS scales and either CSF opioids or β-endorphin. The only correlation approaching significance was a positive one between β-endorphin and the Disinhibition subscale ($r = 0.33$, $p < 0.05$). In terms of pain tolerance, the direction of the latter finding makes sense, since high-sensation-seekers have greater tolerance for painful intensities of stimulation induced by noise, electric shock, and pressure (46). Perhaps the findings of a negative correlation in the Swedish study have something to do with the fact that the subjects were pain patients. This is an area where further exploration is clearly indicated.

Schalling et al. (34) have grouped a number of disorders and extreme personality types under the label "Disinhibitory Psychopathology." Certainly, most drug abusers would be included in this category, defined by the traits of impulsiveness, sensation seeking, and undersocialization. One of their findings in psychopathic criminals (21) is lower levels of urinary cortisol than other prisoners incarcerated in an institution where life was reportedly stressful. Virkkunen (43) has reported similar findings in psychopaths. The personality and biochemical variables in the Ballenger et al. (3) study were subjected to a factor analysis in order to define dimensions of biopsychological interest, and the results were reported in Zuckerman et al. (49). Figure 1 shows the plotted loadings of the variables on factor dimensions I and III. Factor III is a dimension defined by neuroticism at one pole and plasma MHPG at the opposite pole. Factor I is a dimension closely resembling Eysenck's P or Schalling et al.'s Disinhibitory dimension. The highest loading scale on the factor is the SS Disinhibition scale; the SS General, MMPI Hypomania, and EPQ P scales also define the positive pole of the factor. At the negative pole are two biochemical variables: CSF NE and CSF cortisol. Also loading negatively, but not as highly as the other two biochemical variables, are plasma DBH, serum cortisol, and plasma amine oxidase. Since the CSF measures were obtained from a lumbar puncture (LP) and the blood measures were also obtained at about that time, it could be argued that the relationships represent the differential reactions of high and low disinhibitory personalities to the stress or anticipated stress of the procedure. While this state interpretation of the biochemical data still remains a possibility, CSF NE and cortisol did not correlate with a measure of state anxiety obtained just prior to the LP. LPs tend to be one-time procedures that are not compatible with experimental methods.

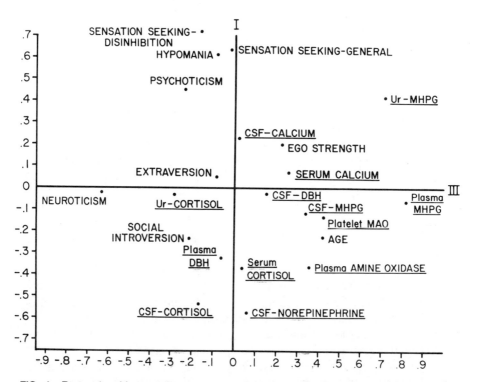

FIG. 1. Factor plot of factors I (Disinhibition) and III (Neuroticism). (From Zuckerman, Ballenger, and Post, ref. 49, with permission.)

FUTURE PROSPECTS

There are two major limitations on the work done to date that links personality, drug abuse, and the psychopharmacology of both. One limitation is the indirect and uncertain indices of brain pharmacology. The other is the correlational nature of most of the research. Do the correlations mean that differences in reactivities of neurotransmitter systems account for differences in personality traits, or is it the other way around? The methodology issue may eventually be solved by the new technologies of PET scanning, which will allow observation of activity of these systems in specific parts of the brain. The localization of activity is important in view of the finding that drugs may increase activity of a neurotransmitter in one area of the brain while decreasing it in another (8). PET research on personality has started at the laboratory of Buchsbaum and Haier (13), using tagged glucose to identify brain activity as glucose is taken up. However, the development of a dopamine-selective PET scan is of immense interest, since the evidence points to the dopaminergic systems as the fundamental mediators of both drive and reward, including the reward effects of many drugs.

The correlational uncertainties of the findings could be resolved by prospective, longitudinal studies of persons at risk for becoming chronic drug abusers. There is already a high-risk group available in most communities: adolescents of ages 13 to 16 who have just begun experimenting with alcohol and marijuana. Few of them will get into hard drugs like cocaine and heroin, but the early identification of those few will tell us much about the biological and social risk factors in addiction. If we used our biological and personality measures with these adolescents, we could test prediction rather than concurrent events. Magnusson (23), for instance, has reported that motor restlessness, rated aggressiveness, *and* low levels of urinary adrenaline at age 13 predicted subsequent adult criminality at ages 18 to 26. This kind of study of high-risk groups has been quite successful in studies of schizophrenia. The danger of longitudinal studies is that one will select the wrong predictor variables at the beginning and therefore fail to predict the outcomes. The current literature on personality and biological correlates of drug abuse can tell us where we should place our bets. All we need is someone to stake us.

REFERENCES

1. Adolfsson, R., Gottfries, L. G., Oreland, L., Roos, B. E., and Winblad, B. (1978): Monoamine oxidase activity and serotogenic turnover in human brain. *Progress in Neuropsychopharmacology,* 2:225–230.
2. Arqué, J., Segurn, R., and Torrubia, B. (1985): *Biochemical Correlates of Sensation Seeking and Susceptibility to Punishment Scales: A Study in Individuals with Somatoform Disorders and Normals.* Paper presented at the Second Annual Meeting of the International Society for the Study of Individual Differences, San Feliu, Spain. June 20–24.
3. Ballenger, J. C., Post, R. M., Jimerson, D. C., Lake, C. R., Murphy, D. L., Zuckerman, M., and Cronin, I. (1983): Biochemical correlates of personality traits in normals: An exploratory study. *Personality Individual Differences,* 4:615–625.

4. Blackburn, R. (1978): Cardiovascular correlates of psychopathy. In: *Psychopathic Behavior: Approaches to Research,* edited by R. D. Hare and D. Schalling, pp. 157–164. Wiley, New York.

5. Carrol, E. N., and Zuckerman, M. (1977): Psychopathology and sensation seeking in 'downers,' 'speeders,' and 'trippers': A study of the relationship between personality and drug choice. *Int. J. Addictions,* 12:591–601.

6. Clavier, R. M., and Gerfen, C. R. (1982): Intracranial self-stimulation in the thalamus of the rat. *Brain Res.,* 8:353–358.

7. Craig, R. J. (1985): *The Personality Structure of Heroin Addicts.* Paper presented at the National Institute on Drug Abuse Technical Review Meeting on Innovative Technologies in Drug Abuse Research, Bethesda, Maryland. October 3.

8. Dworkin, S. I., and Smith, J. E. (1985): *Behavioral Contingencies Involved in Drug-Induced Neurotransmitter Turnover Changes.* Paper presented at the National Institute on Drug Abuse Technical Review Meeting on Innovative Technologies in Drug Abuse Research, Bethesda, Maryland. October 3.

9. Ellison, G. D. (1979): Animal models of psychopathology. In: *Psychopathology in Animals,* edited by J. D. Keegan, pp. 81–101. Academic Press, New York.

10. Emmons, T. D., and Webb, W. W. (1974): Subjective correlates of emotional responsivity and stimulation seeking in psychopaths, normals, and acting-out neurotics. *J. Consult. Clin. Psychol.,* 42:620–625.

11a. Eysenck, H. J., and Eysenck, S. B. G. (1975): *Manual of the Eysenck Personality Questionnaire.* Hodder and Stoughton, London.

11b. Fowler, J. C., von Knorring, L., and Oreland, L. (1980): Platelet monoamine oxidase activity in sensation seekers. *Psychiatr. Res.,* 3:273–279.

12. Freedman, D. X., and Halaris, A. E. (1978): Monoamines and the biochemical mode of action of LSD at synapses. In: *Psychopharmacology: A Generation of Progress,* edited by M. A. Lipton, A. DiMascio, and K. F. Killam, pp. 347–357. Raven Press, New York.

13. Haier, R. J. (1985): *PET and EP Imaging: Differences in Introversion-Extroversion and Sensation Seeking.* Paper presented at the Second Annual Meeting of the International Society for the Study of Individual Differences, San Feliu, Spain. June 20–24.

14. Johansson, F., Almay, B. G. L., von Knorring, L., Terenius, L., and Åström, M. (1979): Personality traits in chronic pain patients related to endorphin levels in cerebrospinal fluid. *Psychiatry Res.,* 1:231–239.

15. Khavari, K. A., Humes, M., and Mabry, E. (1977): Personality correlates of hallucinogen use. *J. Abnorm. Psychol.,* 86:172–178.

16. Kilpatrick, D. G., Sutker, P. B., and Smith, A. D. (1976): Deviant drug and alcohol use: The role of anxiety, sensation seeking and other personality variables. In: *Emotions and Anxiety: New Concepts, Methods and Applications,* edited by M. Zuckerman and C. D. Spielberger, pp. 247–278. Erlbaum, Hillsdale, New Jersey.

17. von Knorring, A. L., Bohman, M., von Knorring, L., and Oreland, L. (1985): Platelet MAO activity as a biological marker in subgroups of alcoholism. *Acta Psychiatr. Scand.,* 72:51–58.

18. von Knorring, L., and Oreland, L. (1985): Personality traits and platelet monoamine oxidase in tobacco smokers. *Psychol. Med.,* 15:327–334.

19. von Knorring, L., Oreland, L., and Winblad, B. (1984): Personality traits related to monoamine oxidase activity in platelets. *Psychiatry Res.,* 12:11–26.

20. Kulcsár, Z., Kutor, L., and Arató, M. (1984): Sensation seeking, its biochemical correlates, and its relation to vestibulo-ocular functions. In: *Personality Psychology in Europe: Theoretical and Empirical Developments,* edited by H. Bonarius, G. van Heck, and N. Smid, pp. 327–346. Swets and Zeitlinger, Lisse, The Netherlands.

21. Levander, S., Mattson, D., Schalling, D., and Dalteg, A.: In: *Psychopathology: An Interactional Perspective,* edited by D. Magnusson and A. Ohman. Academic Press, New York (*in press*).

22. Lidberg, L., Tuck, J. R., Åsberg, M., Scalia-Tombia, G. P., and Bertillson, L. (1985): Homicide, suicide, and CSF 5-HIAA. *Acta Psychiatr. Scand.,* 71:230–236.

23. Magnusson, D. (1985): *Adult Delinquency in the Light of Conduct and Physiology at an Early Age* (Report Supplement 63). Department of Psychology, The University of Stockholm, Sweden.

24. Malatesta, V. J., Sutker, P. B., and Trieber, F. A. (1981): Sensation seeking and chronic public drunkenness. *J. Consult. Clin. Psychol.,* 49:292–294.

25. Mason, S. T. (1984): *Catecholamines and Behavior.* Cambridge University Press, Cambridge.

26. Murphy, D. L., Belmaker, R. H., Buchsbaum, M. S., Martin, N. F., Ciaranello, R., and Wyatt,

R. J. (1977): Biogenic amine related enzymes and personality variations in normals. *Psychol. Med.,* 7:149–157.

27. Okamato, M. (1978): Barbiturates and alcohol: Comparative overviews on neurophysiology and neurochemistry. In: *Psychopharmacology: A Generation of Progress,* edited by M. A. Lipton, A. DiMascio, and K. F. Killam, pp. 1575–1590. Raven Press, New York.

28. Oreland, L., and Fowler, C. (1982): Brain and platelet monoamine oxidase activities in relation to central monoaminergic activity in mice and man. In: *Exerpta Medica International Congress Series, No. 564,* edited by K. Kamijo, E. Usdin, and T. Nagatsu, pp. 312–320. Elsevier, Amsterdam.

29. Perris, C., Eisemann, M., von Knorring, L., Oreland, L., and Perris, H. (1984): Personality traits and monoamine oxidase activity in platelets in depressed patients. *Neuropsychobiology,* 12:201–205.

30. Perris, C., Jacobsson, L., von Knorring, L., Oreland, L., Perris, H., and Ross, S. B. (1980): Enzymes related to biogenic amine metabolism and personality characteristics in depressed patients. *Acta Psychiatr. Scand.,* 61:477–484.

31. Platt, J. J., and Labate, C. (1976): *Heroin Addiction: Theory, Research and Treatment.* Wiley, New York.

32. van Praag, H. M. (1984): Depression, suicide and serotonin metabolism in the brain. In: *Neurobiology of Mood Disorders,* edited by R. M. Post and J. C. Ballenger, pp. 601–618. Williams and Wilkins, Baltimore.

33. Schalling, D., Åsberg, M., and Edman, G. (1984): *Personality and CSF Monoamine Metabolites.* Preliminary manuscript, Department of Psychiatry and Psychology, Karolinska Hospital, and the Department of Psychology, University of Stockholm, Sweden.

34. Schalling, D., Åsberg, M., and Edman, G. (1985): *Personality and Neurochemical Risk Factors for Disinhibitory Psychopathology.* Paper presented at IVth World Congress of Biological Psychiatry, Philadelphia, Pennsylvania. September.

35. Schalling, D., Edman, G., and Åsberg, M. (1983): Impulsive cognitive style and inability to tolerate boredom. In: *Biological Bases of Sensation Seeking, Impulsivity and Anxiety,* edited by M. Zuckerman, pp. 125–147. Erlbaum, Hillsdale, New Jersey.

36. Schooler, C., Zahn, T. P., Murphy, D. L., and Buchsbaum, M. S. (1978): Psychological correlates of monoamine oxidase in normals. *J. Nerv. Ment. Dis.,* 166:177–186.

37. Schwarz, R. M., Burkhart, B. R., and Green, B. (1978): Turning on or turning off: Sensation seeking or tension reduction as motivational determinants of alcohol use. *J. Consult. Clin. Psychol.,* 46:1144–1145.

38. Segal, B. S., Huba, G. J., and Singer, J. F. (1980): *Drugs, Daydreaming, and Personality: A Study of College Youth.* Erlbaum, Hillsdale, New Jersey.

39. Skolnick, N. J., and Zuckerman, M. (1979): Personality change in chronic drug abusers: A comparison of treatment and no-treatment groups. *J. Consult. Clin. Psychol.,* 47:768–770.

40. Soubrié, P. (1986): Reconciling the role of central serotonin neurons in humans and animal behavior. *Behav. Brain Sciences,* 9:319–363.

41. Stein, L. (1978): Reward transmitters: Catecholamines and opioid peptides. In: *Psychopharmacology: A Generation of Progress,* edited by M. A. Lipton, A. DiMascio, and K. F. Killam, pp. 569–581. Raven Press, New York.

42. Umberkoman-Wiita, B., Vogel, W. H., and Wiita, P. J. (1981): Some biochemical and behavioral (sensation seeking) correlates in healthy adults. *Res. Communications Psychol. Psychiatry Behav.,* 6:303–316.

43. Virkkunen, M. (1985): Urinary free cortisol in habitually violent offenders. *Acta Psychiatr. Scand.,* 72:40–44.

44. Wise, R. A. (1980): Action of drugs of abuse on brain reward systems. *Pharmacol. Biochem. Behav.,* 13:213–223.

45. Wise, R. A. (1981): Intracranial self-stimulation: Mapping against the lateral boundaries of the dopaminergic cells of the substantia nigra. *Brain Res.,* 213:190–194.

46. Zuckerman, M. (1979): *Sensation Seeking: Beyond the Optimal Level of Arousal.* Erlbaum, Hillsdale, New Jersey.

47. Zuckerman, M. (1983): Sensation seeking: The initial motive for drug abuse. In: *Etiological Aspects of Alcohol and Drug Abuse,* edited by E. Gotheil, K. A. Druley, T. E. Skoloda, and H. M. Waxman, pp. 202–220. Charles C. Thomas, Springfield, Illinois.

48. Zuckerman, M. (1984): Sensation seeking: A comparative approach to a human trait. *Behav. Brain Sciences,* 7:413–471.

49. Zuckerman, M., Ballenger, J. C., and Post, R. M. (1984): The neurobiology of some dimensions of personality. In: *International Review of Neurobiology, Vol. 25,* edited by J. R. Smythiies and R. J. Bradley, pp. 391–436. Academic Press, New York.
50. Zuckerman, M., Bone, R. N., Neary, R., Mangelsdorff, D., and Brustman, B. (1972): What is the sensation seeker? Personality trait and experience correlates of the Sensation Seeking Scales. *J. Consult. Clin. Psychol.,* 39:308–321.
51. Zuckerman, M., Eysenck, S. B. G., and Eysenck, H. J. (1978): Sensation seeking in England and America: Cross cultural, age and sex comparisons. *J. Consult. Clin. Psychol.,* 46:139–149.
52. Zuckerman, M., Sola, S., Masterson, J., and Angelone, J. V. (1975): MMPI patterns in drug abusers before and after treatment in therapeutic communities. *J. Consult. Clin. Psychol.,* 43: 286–296.

Brain Reward Systems and Abuse, edited by
J. Engel and L. Oreland.
Raven Press, New York © 1987.

Addiction: Clinical and Theoretical Considerations

Nils Bejerot

Department of Social Medicine, Karolinska Institute, S-172 83 Sundbyberg, Sweden

I lack an important component among the chapters from the neurochemical front in this volume: an attempt to give an all-embracing theory on how dependence may be described in general terms. Then, perhaps, we who have worked with drug abusers for decades and feel that we have achieved a clinical familiarity with these paradoxical conditions could attempt to give some theoretical contributions.

First, I would like to say that, from the point of view of social medicine, we must identify several different forms of addiction even to the same drug, for instance, morphine.

Morphinism that arises as a complication to medical treatment differs completely in regard to risk groups, initiation, mechanisms of spread, clinical picture, social complications, treatment and prognosis from the epidemic forms of opiate addiction, where the motive for drug consumption is not relief of pain but primarily a search for intense pleasure. Both these forms differ clinically from the classic opium smoking which in some countries is no great breach of norms. There are also some other forms of opiate dependence (1,2,5,6).

For anyone with a biological education it is clear that the development of dependence is based on pleasurable experiences via the brain reward systems. I do not know of any case where an individual has developed a dependence upon drugs that give unpleasant sensations. The experience of pleasure—or a marked reduction of pain and discomfort—is the basis for an interest in drug consumption. The stronger the experience of pleasure—or amelioration of pain—the more firmly hooked the individual will be. Therefore, different drugs give rise to dependences of differing strength and at a different rate.

The pleasure-producing properties of the drug are thus the basic element. In addition, the size of the dose is important. If it is too low there will be no dependence; if it is too high there may be side effects and complications that overshadow the stimulation of pleasure and counteract the development of dependence. In addition, the means of administration are important for the development of the dynamics of dependence. The sooner after administration the drug effects are experienced, the quicker dependence seems to develop. Oral administration (for injectable drugs) cannot compete with subcutaneous injections, which in their turn cannot compete with intravenous administration. These methods may be superceded, however, by inhalation where the drug can be smoked or sniffed. Administration via a micropipette directly into the brain reward systems should, therefore, give rise to the most rapid development of dependence, on condition that the individual can recognize the significance of administration.

Let me first say a few words on the development of tolerance, a phenomenon that has previously been denoted by the unfortunate term "physical dependence." I consider that tolerance is only an incidental complication that does not affect dependence as such. This may be illustrated in several ways.

If, for instance, we give methadone in food in small but successively rising doses to experimental animals or to people who are not aware of the situation, administration may be raised to saturation level without producing any euphoric effects. Even if the individual in this situation is given large doses of heroin there will be no euphoria. This is the theoretical basis for the clinical "methadone blockade" ad modum Doles and Nyswander (7). If the methadone were suddenly discontinued the usual vegetative abstinence syndrome would naturally develop with great force. On the other hand, if methadone were gradually reduced during a period of about a month, the individual could be detoxicated without discomfort.

In this example, the individual has received up to saturation doses of the drug, has been "physically dependent," but has not developed an addiction because she or he had not experienced any pleasurable sensations. Even if the individual experienced pleasurable sensations, addiction would not have developed unless he or she associated these with the administration of the drug.

If, for instance, a pregnant woman begins to abuse heroin, the fetus receives the drug via the placenta, develops a tolerance as the mother does, and should, of course, experience euphoria when the mother injects the drug. After delivery the child may even die of abstinence reactions if she or he is not detoxicated lege artis. But this newborn individual is still not a drug addict, since the infant cannot associate the pleasurable sensations with drug administration.

Previously, it had been thought that addiction was fundamentally of a pharmacological and physiological nature, but this is evidently a misleading view of dependence. The symptoms that have been studied and described are rather side effects and complications of dependence, which I consider arise from the most primitive form of learning, unconscious conditioning.

We all know people who have developed alcohol addiction, alcoholism, and we are all familiar with the toxic effects that alcohol causes in all the organ systems of the body. Also everyone should be familiar with the well-known phenomenon of nondrinking alcoholics.

Clinically it is well-established that nondrinking alcoholics rapidly relapse into their old drinking pattern if, after decades, they test their trigger mechanism.

These individuals have lost control in regard to drinking, because they have developed an alcohol dependence. The same seems to apply to nicotinists who have not smoked for years: the old consumption pattern is quickly reactivated when they relapse.

There are some circumstances where it can be shown that this learned attachment to drug effects is located in memory. In senile dementia, one sometimes sees how patients suddenly forget that they have been smokers, and then the craving for nicotine and smoking disappears completely. This, in my opinion, is no stranger than that a young man in love, who loses his memory temporarily through a cerebral injury, does not recognize his loved one when she comes to his sick bed. Consequently, he cannot show her any signs of affection: one cannot be in love with a person one has never heard of.

There are a number of clinical conditions where one finds phenomena remarkably similar to nicotinism, alcoholism, and classic drug addiction. Among these are gambling, pyromania, and kleptomania. In strength and endurance all these conditions seem to be close to sexual behavior.

Characteristic of these conditions, which I would call addictions, is that they are highly stereotyped, monotonous, repetitive, strongly emotionally colored, and usually without any biological function except their ability to stimulate the desired pleasure.

It is characteristic of both drug addiction and analogous drug-free conditions that they are very little affected by rational thought. It is as difficult to talk an alcoholic into abstinence as to get a love-sick person to give up an unsuitable partner.

Drug dependence may therefore be described clinically as a deep, chronic love relationship to the pleasant effects of the drug. More theoretically it could be said that drug addiction is a dependence acquired through unconscious conditioning, where the craving for the drug effects has taken on the character and strength of natural drives. It is plausible to assume that in regard to neurophysiology the condition goes back to some extent to the same key structures as sexuality and may be considered as equivalent to this (3,4).

From this point of view it is misleading to call caffeinism, nicotinism, alcoholism, compulsive gambling, pyromania, kleptomania, or sexual aberrations "illnesses." On the other hand, as we know, excessive amounts of alcohol will certainly cause illness, and lack of care in handling sexual drives may lead to all sorts of complications.

It is, however, quite another matter that the complications of dependence interfere with addictive behavior. Health services, however, can only treat these complications, since craving/dependence in itself is like a love relationship and, consequently, not of a medical nature.

The ultimate consequence of this analysis is that health services seem doomed to be counter-productive in regard to the treatment of addicts: it is only the complications (the breaking mechanism) that can be treated and perhaps eliminated. This, however, does not mean that we should moralize over the complications. These we should treat, but modification of destructive or asocial behavior lies outside the sphere of medicine.

The conditions I have hitherto discussed I would call "positive addictions;" in these cases, the individual is driven by a craving for an immediate pleasure reward, often at the cost of long-term loss of pleasure, judged from a total viewpoint (the alcoholic destroys her or his health, financial situation, family, social position, etc.).

It is possible, even probable, that the conditions where an individual obstinately and senselessly tries primarily to avoid or eliminate certain stimuli (phobias, compulsive behavior, nail-biting, neurodermatitis, etc.) also are based on unconscious conditioning. These mirror or inverted conditions, which should then be called "negative addictions," seem to be as little influenced by logical and rational arguments as hate or paranoid reactions.

Love and hate have thousands of different causes, but the strongly fixated, stereotyped, emotionally loaded reactions seem to have been learned through unconscious conditioning and therefore are not particularly susceptible to reason. On the other hand they can be unconditioned, but we should take care not to bring dynamic psychotherapy into the picture. In the end, it is behavioral psychology that might help us to treat all these difficult afflictions where, otherwise, prevention is the all-important approach.

REFERENCES

1. Bejerot, N. (1968): An epidemic of phenmetrazine dependence—Epidemiological and clinical aspects. In: *Adolescent Drug Dependence,* edited by C. W. M. Wilson, pp. 55–66. Pergamon Press, London.
2. Bejerot, N. (1970): *Addiction and Society.* Charles C. Thomas, Springfield, Illinois.
3. Bejerot, N. (1972): *Addiction—An Artificially Induced Drive.* Charles C. Thomas, Springfield, Illinois.
4. Bejerot, N. (1972): A theory of addiction as an artificially induced drive. *Am. J. Psychiatry,* 128: 842–846.
5. Bejerot, N. (1975): Drug abuse and drug policy. An epidemiological and methodological study of drug abuse of intravenous type in the Stockholm Police arrest population 1965–1970 in relation to changes in drug policy. *Acta Psychiatr. Scand.,* Suppl. 256.
6. Bejerot, N. (1980): Addiction to pleasure. A biological and social-psychological theory of addiction. In: *Theories on Drug Abuse. Selected Contemporary Perspectives* (NIDA Research Monograph 30), edited by D. J. Lettieri, M. Sayers, and H. Wallenstein Pearson, pp. 246–255. National Institute on Drug Abuse, Rockville, Maryland.
7. Dole, V., and Nyswander, M. (1973): A medical treatment for Diacetylmorphine (heroin). Addiction: A clinical trial with methadone. In: *Methadone: Experiences and Issues,* edited by C. D. Chambers and L. Brill, pp. 53–65. Behavioral Publications, New York.

Brain Reward Systems and Abuse, edited by
J. Engel and L. Oreland.
Raven Press, New York © 1987.

Alcohol Consumption, Dependence, and Central Norepinephrine Metabolism in Humans

Stefan Borg, Paula Liljeberg, and Dick Mossberg

*Karolinska Institute, Department of Psychiatry, at St. Göran's Hospital,
S-112 81 Stockholm, Sweden*

The importance of the central noradrenergic system for the actions of ethanol has been demonstrated in several animal studies. For example, greater intoxicating effects have been reported after norepinephrine depletion in animals, indicating a connection with tolerance (23). The reinforcing effects of ethanol have been prevented by enzyme inhibition of norepinephrine synthesis (12,16). Increased alcohol consumption in a free-choice situation has been reported after depletion of the dorsal noradrenergic pathways of the brain (23,24). The hypothesis was put forward that ethanol intake was one way to increase norepinephrine turnover in the CNS.

One way to study central nervous noradrenergic metabolism in living subjects under different clinical conditions has been to measure norepinephrine and/or its main metabolite, 3-methoxy-4-hydroxy-phenylethyleneglycol (HMPG, or MOPEG) in the lumbar cerebrospinal fluid (CSF).

It has been assumed that the concentration of HMPG at least partly reflects the activity of the central noradrenergic system (13). An increase of the functional activity of the central norepinephrine neurons has been shown to lead to an increased release of norepinephrine, resulting in elevated HMPG levels in the tissue (14).

A significant correlation has been reported between the HMPG concentrations in several brain areas, cisternal CSF, and plasma in primates (18).

However, the exact relationship between HMPG levels in the CSF and cerebral norepinephrine activity is unclear. A high correlation between plasma and CSF levels of HMPG in patients with high peripheral norepinephrine production indicates that a substantial portion of the HMPG can be derived from the plasma (25).

In a series of studies, male alcoholic patients were investigated under different clinical conditions and compared with healthy controls. The HMPG level in the CSF was determined with high specifity and accuracy with the aid of gas chromatography and mass spectrometry (6–11,33).

Patients were studied during acute intoxication, acute withdrawal, after 1 and 3 weeks of abstinence in the hospital, and after long-term abstinence. The latter group was followed with clinical ratings three times a week for 6 months. Clinical conditions were measured using items from the Comprehensive Psychopathological Rating Scale (CPRS) and additional items focusing on craving (27,28).

Results of the clinical ratings are shown in Fig. 1. After a period of abuse the

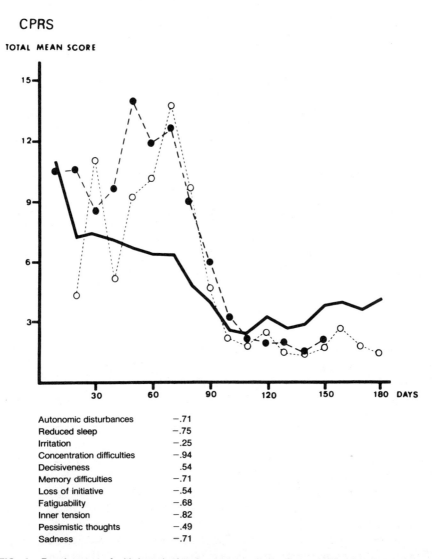

FIG. 1. Development of withdrawal-related symptoms during long-term abstinence in a group of alcoholic patients. Mean score for 10-day periods of the whole group and two individual cases. Correlation between individual items and duration of abstinence. *Open circles,* subject A; *filled circles,* subject B; *solid line,* mean of the whole group.

score for withdrawal-related items was high, and a rapid decrease was seen during the first 2 weeks of abstinence. Thereafter, a gradual decrease of the withdrawal-related items was seen for about 2 to 3 months, indicating a gradual disappearance of a protracted withdrawal syndrome. In studying the affective state of the patients (Fig. 2), depressive as well as elevated periods of mood were registered (CPRS items > 1.0 in variables for depression and euphoria, respectively). This pattern was seen in most of the patients in spite of the fact that no one exhibited or reported affective illness before entering the study. Relapses have been reported to occur shortly after both types of periods (30).

Figure 3 summarizes the results of the HMPG levels in the CSF for different clinical groups studied. High levels of HMPG were found during intoxication, and the HMPG levels of the CSF were significantly correlated to blood ethanol concentrations ($r = 0.49$; $p < 0.05$) (11). Levels were somewhat lower during acute withdrawal than during intoxication but still significantly elevated compared to healthy controls. The HMPG levels in the CSF were significantly correlated to a number of clinical withdrawal symptoms, such as diastolic blood pressure ($r = 0.21$; $p < 0.05$), pulse rate ($r = 0.35$; $p < 0.001$), visual hallucinations ($r = 0.22$; $p < 0.05$), sleeping disorders ($r = 0.35$; $p < 0.01$), trembling ($r = 0.24$; $p < 0.05$) and restlessness ($r = 0.25$; $p < 0.05$).

A negative correlation was established between HMPG levels and craving for alcohol ($r = 0.26$; $p < 0.02$) (7).

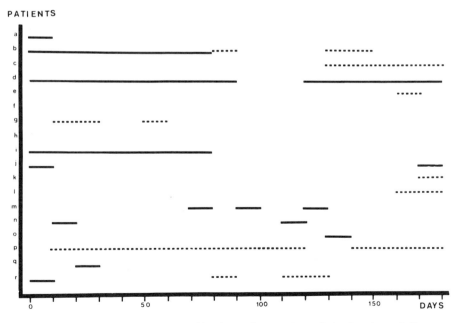

FIG. 2. Periods with elevated mood and/or depressive symptoms during long-term abstinence in alcohol-dependent patients. Mean values > 1.0 of 10-day periods for pessimistic thoughts and elevated mood respectively.

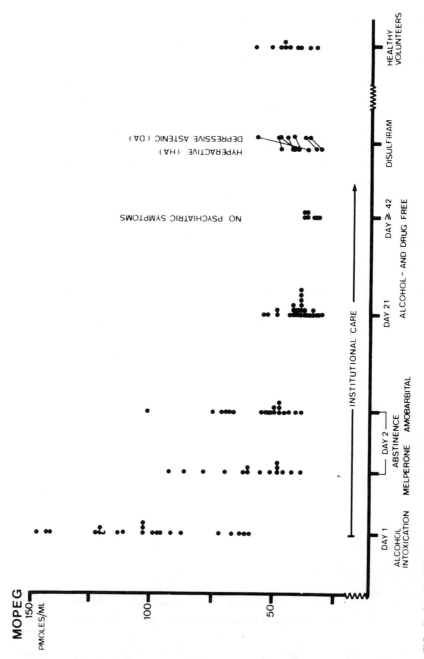

FIG. 3. Levels of 3-methoxy-4-hydroxy-phenylethyleneglycol (MOPEG or HMPG) in the CSF of alcohol-dependent patients during different clinical conditions.

In alcoholic patients abstinent for more than 6 weeks and without psychiatric symptoms, subnormal levels of HMPG were seen (8). In those patients investigated during both elevated and depressed mood states, levels of HMPG were lower during elevated than during depressed periods (6,28). A significant negative correlation was seen between HMPG levels and craving, as was noted during acute withdrawal.

A group of healthy male controls was studied for comparison. All had been alcohol-free for at least 1 week before lumbar puncture. As can be seen in Fig. 4, a significant correlation was found between low HMPG levels and high long-term alcohol consumption. Controls with first-degree relatives with alcohol problems had significantly lower HMPG levels than the others (10). Thus, in healthy controls, as well, it was possible to associate low HMPG levels with high long-term alcohol consumption. The finding of low levels in subjects with first-degree relatives with alcohol problems also indicates that a genetic factor may play a role.

In one experiment, lumbar punctures were performed in connection with the intake of 60 to 120 g of ethanol per os (9,11). The experiment was performed in the same way but without ethanol intake 1 week before or after to establish baseline conditions. Lumbar punctures were performed during acute intoxication, and results were compared to those of alcohol patients examined during acute intoxication and after 1 week of abstinence. As seen in Fig. 5, a significant

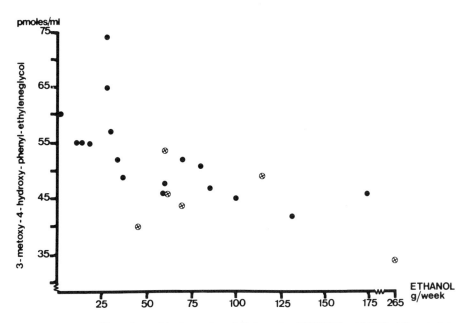

FIG. 4. Levels of 3-methoxy-4-hydroxy-phenylethyleneglycol (MOPEG or HMPG) at 8 pm in the CSF of healthy males in relation to long-term alcohol consumption. *Open circles with X,* volunteers with first-degree relatives with alcohol problems.

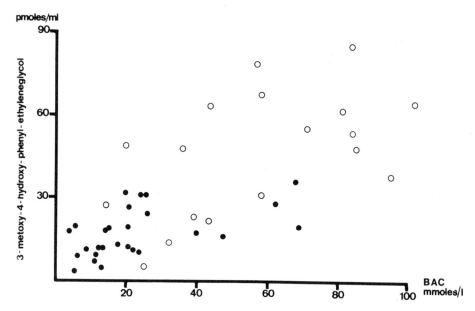

FIG. 5. Changes of 3-methoxy-4-hydroxy-phenylethyleneglycol (MOPEG or HMPG) in the CSF of alcohol intake in relation to blood alcohol concentration (BAC) in intoxicated alcoholic patients (*open circles*) and healthy volunteers (*filled circles*).

correlation was noted between blood ethanol concentration and HMPG elevations. However, when a comparison was made between alcoholics and controls, separate regression lines were observed between the groups. HMPG levels in the healthy subjects never reached the levels that could be noted in the patients. The experiments thus support the notion that ethanol increases HMPG levels and indicate possible differences in the noradrenergic systems of alcoholics and non-alcoholics. The alcoholics seem to be able to respond to increased concentrations of ethanol with increased HMPG stimulation when blood ethanol concentrations are very high. Normal consumers can only respond up to a certain HMPG level after which no further HMPG elevation is possible despite still higher ethanol concentrations.

Assuming that HMPG levels in the CSF reflect central noradrenergic activity, a correlation between low noradrenergic activity and high alcohol consumption was seen in nonalcoholic subjects. The finding that subjects with first-degree relatives with alcohol problems had lower HMPG levels is in line with the assumption that a genetic factor is of importance for the HMPG levels and possibly also the noradrenergic activity resulting in high alcohol consumption. Signs of low noradrenergic activity were also seen in alcoholics but were not observed unless they had been without access to alcohol for several weeks. This might be explained by the fact that the alcohol withdrawal syndrome is associated with an increased noradrenergic activity—indicated, among other things, by the correlation between HMPG levels and several withdrawal symptoms—and that the protracted withdrawal syndrome was observed for 2 to 3 months after alcohol intake had stopped. The assumption of a connection between low noradrenergic activity and high alcohol consumption was also strengthened by the observation that low noradrenergic activity indicated by low HMPG levels in the CSF was linked to subjective feelings of craving for alcohol in alcoholics.

These findings are in line with the hypothesis put forward by Kiianmaa (23) that alcohol intake is a way for the individual to increase noradrenergic activity.

The observation of periods with elevated and depressed mood during long-term abstinence indicates an affective dysregulation in alcoholics. Whether this precedes or is a consequence of abuse is a question that cannot be determined in these studies. A connection between alcoholism and some affective disorders has been reported in family and epidemiological studies (2,22,34). A connection between hyperactivity and alcoholism has also been reported (1,5,29). A connection between affective dysregulation in alcoholics and central noradrenergic activity is indicated by the observation of lower HMPG levels during elevated than during depressed states. In primates, low norepinephrine concentrations in the CSF were reported to be associated with the most severe responses to social separation (26). In humans, low HMPG levels in urine have been reported in hyperactive children (31,37), and depressed states have been coupled to aberrant noradrenergic activity (15,17,36), indicating connections between noradrenergic systems and hyperactivity as well as affective disorders.

The interpretation of increased levels of HMPG in the CSF during alcohol intoxication is complicated by the fact that HMPG levels in the periphery are increased due to the redox shift induced by ethanol (34). Some of the HMPG found in the CSF could therefore be expected to originate from the periphery.

However, the transport of HMPG from plasma into the CSF seems to be rather slow and only a few percent seems to have penetrated after 2 to 4 hr. HMMA (4-hydroxy-3-methoxy-mandelic acid) was measured simultaneously in alcoholic patients and only small amounts were found, which makes it unlikely that most of the HMPG is metabolized to HMMA (32). This supports the contention that there is a connection between HMPG elevations in the CSF and central noradrenergic activity during acute intoxication as well.

Several reports are in line with the assumption that ethanol stimulates noradrenergic activity in humans. High norepinephrine levels of the CSF have been reported after alcohol intoxication (21,32). The same conclusion of increased norepinephrine turnover after alcohol intake has been drawn from experiments with infusions of labeled norepinephrine in human subjects (20).

The observation of high HMPG levels during withdrawal and hangover and the correlation between HMPG levels and different withdrawal signs and symptoms lends support to the assumption of a relationship between increased central norepinephrine activity and symptoms of withdrawal. The observation that the α-agonist clonidine, which reduces noradrenergic turnover, is effective in treating acute alcohol withdrawal is also in line with this hypothesis (4).

When comparing increases of HMPG levels in the CSF during intoxication, alcohol patients seemed to respond in a more active way than nonalcoholics. Thus, low noradrenergic activity might be one factor for an increased norepinephrine stimulation by ethanol. In primates, subjects with low norepinephrine levels in the CSF were reported to respond with a higher norepinephrine increase during ethanol intoxication, supporting this hypothesis (26).

The mechanisms by which ethanol interacts with noradrenergic systems are not known. Chronic ethanol ingestion for 2 months has been reported to lead to a decrease in the density of the β-adrenergic receptor during withdrawal in animal studies (3). French et al. (19), measuring cAMP accumulation, have reported subsensitivity during long-term intoxication and supersensitivity during acute withdrawal. In this way, ethanol seems to have effects similar to those of antidepressive pharmaceuticals (35).

To summarize, our studies are in line with a hypothesis of a connection between alcohol abuse and certain behavioral criteria, e.g., hyperactive and/or affective syndromes, and suggest that low central noradrenergic activity might be one link between alcohol abuse and such conditions. Alcohol intake stimulates noradrenergic activity, and alcoholics may respond to alcohol in a more active way than nonalcoholics, possibly due to differences in the basal noradrenergic activity either of genetic origin or induced by long-term ethanol consumption. This response might be of importance for regulation of affective symptoms as well as intoxication, withdrawal symptoms, and reinforcing effects of ethanol.

REFERENCES

1. Alterman, A. I., and Tarter, R. E. (1983): The transmission of psychological vulnerability: Implications for alcoholism etiology. *J. Nerv. Ment. Dis.,* 171:147–154.
2. Angst, J. (1972): Genetic aspects of depression. In: *Depressive Illness,* edited by P. Kielholz, pp. 28–36. Hans Huber, Basel.
3. Banarjee, S., Sharma, V., and Khanna, J. (1978): Alteration in beta-adrenergic receptor binding during ethanol withdrawal. *Nature,* 276:407–408.
4. Björkqvist, S. E. (1975): Clonidine in alcohol withdrawal. *Acta Psychiatr. Scand.,* 52:256–263.
5. Blouin, A. G. A., Bornstein, R. A., and Trites, R. L. (1978): Teenage alcohol among hyperactive children: A five year follow-up study. *J. Pediatr. Psychol.,* 3:188–194.
6. Borg, S. (1986): Central nervous system noradrenaline metabolism and alcohol consumption in man. *Acta Psychiatr. Scand.,* 73(Suppl. 327):43–60.
7. Borg, S., Czarnecka, A., Kvande, H., Mossberg, D., and Sedvall, G. (1983): Clinical conditions and concentrations of MOPEG in the cerebrospinal fluid and urine of male alcoholic patients during withdrawal. *Alcoholism (NY),* 7:411–415.
8. Borg, S., Kvande, H., Mossberg, D., and Sedvall, G. (1983): Central nervous noradrenaline metabolism in alcoholics during long-term abstinence. *Alcohol Alcohol.,* 18:3.
9. Borg, S., Kvande, H., Mossberg, D., and Valverius, P. (1984): Central noradrenaline metabolism during alcohol intoxication in man—Relationship to blood alcohol concentration. In: *Catecholamines: Neuropharmacology and Central Nervous System—Theoretical Aspects,* edited by E. Usdin, A. Carlsson, A. Dahlström, and J. Engel. pp. 153–157. Alan R. Liss, New York.
10. Borg, S., Kvande, H., Mossberg, D., Valverius, P., and Sedvall, G. (1983): Central nervous system noradrenaline metabolism and alcohol consumption in man. *Pharmacol. Biochem. Behav.,* 18: 375–378.

11. Borg, S., Kvande, H., and Sedvall, G. (1981): Central norepinephrine metabolism during alcohol intoxication in addicts and healthy volunteers. *Science,* 213:1135–1137.
12. Brown, Z. W., Amit, Z., Levitan, D. E., Ögren, S.-O., and Sutherland, E. A. (1977): Noradrenergic mediation of the positive reinforcing properties of ethanol. *Arch. Int. Pharmacodyn. Ther.,* 230: 76–82.
13. Chase, T. N., Gordon, E. K., and Ng, L. K.-Y. (1973): Norepinephrine metabolism in the central nervous system of man. Studies using 3-methoxy-4-hydroxyphenylethylene glycol levels in cerebrospinal fluid. *J. Neurochem.,* 21:581.
14. Crawley, J. N., Roth, R. H., and Maas, J. W. (1979): Locus coeruleus stimulation increases noradrenergic metabolite levels in rat spinal cord. *Brain Res.,* 166:180–184.
15. Curtis, C. G., Cleghorn, R. A., and Sourkes, T. L. (1960): The relationship between affect and the excretion of adrenaline, noradrenaline, and 17-hydroxycorticosteroids. *J. Psychosom. Res.,* 4:176–184.
16. Davis, W. M., Smith, S. G., and Werner, T. E. (1978): Noradrenergic role in the self-administration of ethanol. *Pharmacol. Biochem. Behav.,* 9:369–374.
17. Deneker, S. J., Hägendal, J., and Malmo, U. (1966): Noradrenaline content of cerebrospinal fluid in mental diseases. *Lancet,* 2:754.
18. Elsworth, J. D., Roth, J. H., Stogin, J. M., Leahy, D. J., Moore, M. R., and Redmond, D. E. (1980): Peripheral correlates of central noradrenergic activity. *Society for Neuroscience Abstracts,* 6:140.
19. French, S. W., Palmer, D. S., Narold, M. E., Reid, P. E., and Ramey, C. W. (1975): Noradrenergic sensitivity of the cerebral cortex after chronic ethanol ingestion and withdrawal. *J. Pharmacol. Exp. Ther.,* 194:319–326.
20. Gitlow, S. E., Bertani, L. M., Dziedzic, S. W., and Wong, B. L. (1976): The influence of ethanol upon human catecholamine metabolism. *Ann. N.Y. Acad. Sci.,* 273:263–279.
21. Hawley, R. J., Major, L. F., Schulman, E. A., and Lake, C. R. (1981): CSF levels of norepinephrine during alcohol withdrawal. *Arch. Neurol.,* 38:289–292.
22. Helgason, T. (1964): Epidemiology of mental disorders in Iceland. *Acta Psychiatr. Scand. [Suppl.],* 173:258.
23. Kiianmaa, K. (1980): Alcohol intake and ethanol intoxication in the rat: Effects of a 6-OHOA induced lesion of the ascending noradrenaline pathways. *Eur. J. Pharmacol.,* 64:9–13.
24. Kiianmaa, K., Fuxe, K., Jensen, G., and Ahtee, L. (1975): Evidence for involvement of central NA neurons in alcohol intake. Increased alcohol consumption after degeneration of the NA pathway to the cortex cerebri. *Neurosci. Lett.,* 1:41–45.
25. Kopin, I., Gordon, E. K., Jimerson, D. C.,·and Polinsky, R. J. (1983): Relation between plasma and cerebrospinal fluid levels of 3-methoxy-4-hydroxyphenylethyleneglycol. *Science,* 219:73–75.
26. Kraemer, G. W., Lake, C. R., Ebert, M. H., and McKinney, W. T. (1985): Effects of alcohol on cerebrospinal fluid norepinephrine in rhesus monkeys. *Psychopharmacology (Berlin),* 85:444–448.
27. Liljeberg, P., Mossberg, D., and Borg, S. (1986): Clinical conditions and central noradrenergic activity in long-term abstinent alcoholic patients (*in preparation*).
28. Liljeberg, P., Mossberg, D., and Borg, S. (1986): Clinical conditions during long-term abstinence in alcohol dependent patients with special regard to protracted withdrawal, affective state and clinical symptoms prior to relapse (*in preparation*).
29. Mendelson, W., Johnson, N., and Stewart, M. (1971): Hyperactive children as teenagers: A follow-up study. *J. Nerv. Ment. Dis.,* 153:273–279.
30. Mossberg, D., Liljeberg, P., and Borg, S. (1985): Clinical conditions in alcoholics during long-term abstinence: A descriptive, longitudinal treatment study. *Alcohol,* 2:551–553.
31. Shekim, W. O., Javaid, J., Davis, J. M., and Bylund, D. B. (1983): Urinary MHPG and HVA excretion in boys with attention deficit disorder and hyperactivity treated with d-amphetamine. *Biol. Psychiatry,* 18:707–714.
32. Sjöquist, B., Borg, B., and Kvande, H. (1981): Catecholamine derived compounds in urine and cerebrospinal fluid from alcoholics during and after long-standing intoxication. *Subst. Alcohol Actions Misuse,* 2:63–72.
33. Swahn, D.-G., Sandgärde, B., Wiesel, F.-A., and Sedvall, G. (1976): Simultaneous determination of the three major monoamine metabolites in brain tissue and body fluids by a massfragmentographic method. *Psychopharmacology (Berlin),* 48:147.

34. Winokour, G., Cadoret, R., Dorzab, J., and Baker, M. (1971): Depressive disease, a genetic study. *Arch. Gen. Psychiatry,* 24:135–144.
35. Wolfe, B. B., Harden, T. K., Sporn, J. R., and Molinoff, P. B. (1978): Presynaptic modulation of beta-adrenergic receptors in rat cerebral cortex after treatment with antidepressants. *J. Pharmacol. Exp. Ther.,* 207:446–457.
36. Wyatt, R. J., Portnoy, B., Kupfer, D. J., Snyder, F., and Engelman, K. (1971): Resting plasma catecholamine concentrations in patients with depression and anxiety. *Arch. Gen. Psychiatry,* 24:65–70.
37. Yy-cun, S., and Yu-feng, W. (1984): Urinary 3-methoxy-4-hydroxy-phenylglycol sulfate excretion in seventy-three schoolchildren with minimal brain dysfunction syndrome. *Biol. Psychiatry,* 19: 861–870.

Subject Index

DATE DUE